The Dementia Manifesto

D1447648

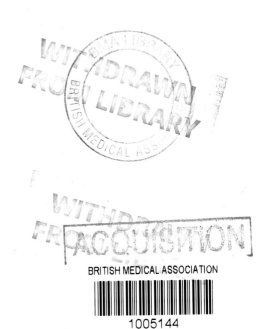

Endorsements for *The Dementia Manifesto*

"I welcome this book which sits squarely alongside my lived experience of dementia and underlines its complexities that are so often overlooked. I wholeheartedly commend the authors' bravery in applying their wisdom and experience to a book which will, I am sure, contribute towards positive change. Indeed, that should be the function of any manifesto worthy of the label. The book is challenging, but so is attempting to live well with dementia, and without challenge nothing will move forwards. This book is a very significant step in the right direction."

Keith Oliver Alzheimer's Society Ambassador, Kent and Medway NHS and Social Care Partnerships Trust (KMPT) Dementia Service User Envoy

"I loved the case vignettes – true to life, rich in narrative detail, precisely constructed and thoughtfully teased apart to illustrate the application of Values-based practice (VBP) in dementia.

The Dementia Manifesto is in essence a comprehensive and heartfelt refutation of an old idea that dementia represents a loss of personhood. Instead, it proclaims as its first principle: Dementia is a unique touchstone for understanding our humanity.

This book describes the principles of Values-based practice in dementia, as an essential complement to Evidence-based practice, and deeply rooted in the established perspectives – philosophical, scientific, ethical, political, legal, institutional – which shape the thinking of practitioners in the field. Key concepts in VBP include the recognition that 'objective facts' are nearly always entangled with values, and the idea of Dissensus – respectful appreciation of the variety of legitimate values at work – as a practical way forward when consensus is impossible."

Dr Catherine Oppenheimer, Oxford

"In *The Dementia Manifesto*, Hughes and Williamson recognize dementia as a human condition that challenges people to find the 'better angels of our nature' and, thereby, never to lose sight of the fact that it is a person who is experiencing what is called dementia. They demonstrate convincingly why it is utterly crucial to recognize that our understanding of dementia and the psychological, social, and pharmacological treatment of people so diagnosed are laden with values and that absent a clear, focused understanding and practice of those values, we shall be treasonous to 'the better angels of our nature'. The case examples they present illustrate wonderfully the complex value-laden interpersonal relationships that people diagnosed and their care partners experience, their respective rights, and the great sensitivity required to understand people in their totality so as to provide optimal person-centred care, or Values-Based Practice, in the authors' terms. The values in and the value of human life demand nothing less. Indeed, they behove us to pay especially close attention to what Hughes and Williamson put forth in this volume."

Steven R. Sabat, Ph.D., FGSA
Professor Emeritus of Psychology, Georgetown University,
Washington, D.C.
Associate Editor, *Dementia: The International Journal of*
Social Research and Practice

"This book makes a timely and unique contribution to the dementia discourse. It brings together theoretical, ethical and practice based knowledge to make the case for a values driven manifesto for people living with dementia. It is infused with a clear commitment to rights and person centredness and foregrounds the importance of relationships, both formal and family and friends, in enhancing well being and personhood. Using vignettes the authors thoughtfully and skilfully illustrate the role and capacity of a values based approach to shift the fulcrum of care towards meaningful, respectful and individualised engagement with different and varied lived experiences of dementia. The book is exquisitely written and captures the reader immediately; it will have wide and refreshing appeal.

The authors bring their considerable clinical, policy and research related expertise and knowledge to bear in an imaginative and coherent text that offer a new lens on how we think and conceptualise dementia and support people living with dementia."

Dr Alisoun Milne
Professor of Social Gerontology and Social Work, University of Kent

The Dementia Manifesto

Putting Values-Based Practice to Work

Julian C. Hughes
University of Bristol

Toby Williamson
University of West London

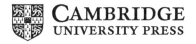

CAMBRIDGE
UNIVERSITY PRESS

CAMBRIDGE
UNIVERSITY PRESS

University Printing House, Cambridge CB2 8BS, United Kingdom

One Liberty Plaza, 20th Floor, New York, NY 10006, USA

477 Williamstown Road, Port Melbourne, VIC 3207, Australia

314–321, 3rd Floor, Plot 3, Splendor Forum, Jasola District Centre, New Delhi – 110025, India

79 Anson Road, #06-04/06, Singapore 079906

Cambridge University Press is part of the University of Cambridge.

It furthers the University's mission by disseminating knowledge in the pursuit of education, learning, and research at the highest international levels of excellence.

www.cambridge.org
Information on this title: www.cambridge.org/9781107535992
DOI: 10.1017/9781316336229

First published 2019

Printed and bound in Great Britain by Clays Ltd, Elcograf S.p.A.

A catalogue record for this publication is available from the British Library.

ISBN 978-1-107-53599-2 Paperback

Cambridge University Press has no responsibility for the persistence or accuracy of URLs for external or third-party internet websites referred to in this publication and does not guarantee that any content on such websites is, or will remain, accurate or appropriate.

Every effort has been made in preparing this book to provide accurate and up-to-date information that is in accord with accepted standards and practice at the time of publication. Although case histories are drawn from actual cases, every effort has been made to disguise the identities of the individuals involved. Nevertheless, the authors, editors, and publishers can make no warranties that the information contained herein is totally free from error, not least because clinical standards are constantly changing through research and regulation. The authors, editors, and publishers therefore disclaim all liability for direct or consequential damages resulting from the use of material contained in this book. Readers are strongly advised to pay careful attention to information provided by the manufacturer of any drugs or equipment that they plan to use.

Julian dedicates this book to
his wife
Anne
with love and gratitude.
Toby dedicates this book to
his wife and his mum
Jane and Karina,
and to family and friends, past and present,
with love and gratitude.
Together we dedicate this book to
all those people,
especially those we have known,
who live and have lived with dementia
and to those who support or have supported them.
For people living with dementia today and in the
future and those who support them,
we hope it contributes to their rights as citizens
and sustains their wishes, feelings, beliefs, and values
as people,
and their lives as human beings and members of
society.

Contents

Contents

Foreword

When Julian Hughes and Toby Williamson approached me about their plans for a Values-based dementia manifesto I was initially sceptical. A timely editorial, perhaps, I wondered, or maybe a 'thought piece' for an academic journal, but was there really a whole book in this?

Just how wrong I was is evident throughout this inspiring and highly original work. From its thoughtful theoretical underpinnings, through a series of insightful chapters on key aspects of dementia care, to its clear conclusions, Hughes and Williamson's *Manifesto* consistently comes good on its promissory subtitle in *Putting Values-Based Practice to Work*.

There is much talk nowadays about 'values based this' and 'values based that'. We are all required to have and to evince 'the right values'. But the Values-based Practice underpinning Hughes and Williamson's Manifesto is not of this kind. It is rather about building the skills and other resources required to support balanced decision making where, as in living with dementia, the operative values are complex and conflicting.

As developed recently in Oxford, the focus of Values-based Practice, so conceived, has been on areas of acute clinical care such as surgery and radiology. Hughes and Williamson's Manifesto brilliantly extends Values-based Practice to the perhaps even greater challenges presented by long-term complex conditions. They are the first to do this. Page after page illustrates how Values-based Practice supports working with people living with dementia, those with dementia and their carers, in ways that are both humane and at the same time deeply practical.

But there is more even than this in their book. In working out the implications of Values-based Practice for dementia care, Hughes and Williamson have greatly enhanced our understanding of Values-based Practice itself. Human Rights are a case in point. In marking itself out as a process- rather than outcomes-focused way of working with values, Values-based Practice has sometimes ended up appearing to be anti-ethics. Hughes and Williamson's nuanced use of Human Rights principles (derived from disability studies), working always alongside the personalisation of decision-making supported by Values-based Practice, nicely exemplifies the essential complementarity between these two approaches.

There is thus no one-size-fits-all when it comes to working with values. The challenges of dementia care illustrate the vital importance of being ready to draw appropriately on the full range of resources available from the 'values tool kit'. The significance of the tool kit runs indeed well beyond the remit of the Manifesto. In highlighting the importance for dementia of rights alongside values, the Manifesto innovatively links these to wider notions of personhood and citizenship. Hughes and Williamson's Values-based Dementia Manifesto thus becomes a touchstone for understanding the human condition as a whole.

Bill (KWM) Fulford
St Catherine's College, Oxford
November 2018

Preface

We all see dementia as a challenge. Indeed, many are frightened by the very prospect of it. This is not unreasonable, because more of us throughout the world are getting it as we live longer. And it's a serious and sometimes devastating condition. The biology and psychology of dementia, its medical and behavioural management, are all dealt with elsewhere. In this book we want to pause to reflect on other aspects of dementia because, as we shall argue, despite everything else about it, dementia is also a way of seeing more clearly the human condition. In the face of a threat to our lives and to our standing as persons with relationships and a sense of dignity and worth, we would argue that it's quite natural to ponder on some of the deeper aspects of our being in, or engagement with, the world. These ponderings are pertinent to us all, not just to those of us who will get or are already living with dementia.

Moreover, there is a particular aspect of the human condition which we wish to consider. It is the pervasiveness of values and the implications of this for dementia and for dementia care in particular. The challenge of the human condition is, in part, the challenge of living out our values in a world of diverse values. Values-based practice (VBP), the topic covered by this series of books, is all about negotiating the world of values. In the context of dementia, it is also a way – amongst other ways – of understanding what we are doing and why: a way to work out what might be for the best. Given that dementia and the problems it can throw up will elicit different value judgements, thinking about dementia can give us a particular values-based way of seeing the world. But seeing the world in this light, as a world replete with intersecting, converging, and diverging values, is also to see dementia differently. It's not solely a condition (and it would be odd given the reality of the human condition if this were the case) describable by facts: dementia is shot through with evaluative judgements.

The new view of dementia, the person-values perspective, enables us to see dementia differently, but, more importantly, it helps us to approach some well-recognized problems associated with living with dementia afresh. In order to do this, we cannot be sectarian. We have to grasp the whole of what it is to be a human person living in the world. This includes, then, the reality of our physical state – a physical state which is at risk of (and will inevitably succumb to) disease. Dementia is a disease which needs to be understood at a pathophysiological level. The biology and relevant pharmacology of dementia are important. But dementia is also a disability with which people live. And people with disabilities have rights as citizens to expect certain sorts of regard. They must be treated; but this treatment is not primarily (foundationally one might say) biomedical treatment, nor indeed is it simply a matter of adding in psychosocial treatment. At a foundational level, it's the treatment that we all expect and deserve as citizens: treatment with respect and courtesy as free people bound together by the deep ties of humanity. The interconnections and interdependencies that constitute our solidarity are preserved in the citizenship of people who live with dementia. Furthermore, this citizenship provides us all with rights. So our standing in the world as citizens is shot through with rights, just as it provides a scaffold for the richness of our shared and diverse values.

This book, we hope, will make explicit how useful a VBP approach can be for dementia care. In part, this will be achieved by showing the pervasiveness of values. In addition, it will be achieved by looking at the particularities of cases. We shall show how the
VBP framework fits and is beneficial in considering different issues in dementia care.
These will include issues around relationships and team work, as well as around diagnosis, behaviour that challenges, truth telling, the end of life, legal matters, communication,
stigma, and social policy, to name but a few. In addition, however, we shall show how
VBP must be cognizant of, and work in partnership with, the rights-based approach to
dementia which emphasizes our standing as citizens.

So dementia – living with dementia and helping others to live well with dementia –
and all of the challenges that go with dementia can be usefully approached via VBP. At
the same time we must keep in mind both the standing of dementia as a disease and its
standing as a disability to which the rights of citizens attach. Meanwhile, by understanding the contribution of VBP to dementia, as well as how the challenge that dementia
poses can enhance VBP, we can understand something more about the human condition.
Our Manifesto is that we should understand dementia as epitomizing the human condition, as both a disease and a disability, and as a reality for which VBP presents a practical
approach bolstered by rights. Moreover, seeing dementia as value-laden, as we must if
we see the human condition aright, makes VBP a natural path to follow in trying to deal
with the moral, legal, social, and political issues that arise in connection with dementia. If
this book achieves even a small part of this ambition, then we shall be able to claim that
it has sparked a revolution, perhaps only at an individual level, but with the potential to
revolutionize our whole approach to dementia.

Acknowledgements

We would like to express our sincere gratitude to the following:

First and foremost, Bill Fulford for his support and encouragement. It's true that without him this book would not have been written, but more than that, he has remained a guide, inspiration, and friend to both.

Colleagues at the Collaborating Centre for Values-Based Practice in Health and Social Care, St Catherine's College, University of Oxford.

Everyone who made suggestions and commented on early drafts of the book, especially:

Reinhard Guss
Philly Hare
Keith and Rosemary Oliver
Camilla Parker
Chris Roberts and Jayne Goodrick.

Barbara Pointon for giving her permission to use her Web of Care diagram in Chapter 12.

Moth Broyles for administrative assistance to Julian.

Catherine Barnes, Kirsten Bot, Jessica Papworth, Neil Ryan, and their colleagues at Cambridge University Press for their patience and encouragement.

Toby would like to express his deepest thanks to Julian for agreeing to co-author this book in the first place; his idea of making it a manifesto; his expertise, experience, advice, comments, and support; and his willingness to see it through to completion.

Julian would like to thank Toby for his unwavering tolerance, fairness, common sense, inspiration, perception, and the knowledge and many insights that he has conveyed through the process of writing this book, and for being such a pleasure to work with.

Authors' Note

All the people featured in the vignettes in this book are fictional but are based upon the authors' collected experience of working with people with dementia, family carers, and practitioners.

Abbreviations

ACP	Advance care planning
AD	Alzheimer's disease
ADRT	Advance decision to refuse treatment
aMCI	Amnestic mild cognitive impairment
ANH	Artificial nutrition and hydration
CPN	Community psychiatric nurse
CPR	Cardiopulmonary resuscitation
CSF	Cerebrospinal fluid
DEEP	Dementia Engagement and Empowerment Project
DLB	Dementia with Lewy bodies
DoLS	Deprivation of Liberty Safeguards
DOR	Dementia-orientated reality
EBM	Evidence-based medicine
EBP	Evidence-based practice
ECHR	European Convention on Human Rights
GP	General practitioner
LPA	Lasting power of attorney
MCA	Mental Capacity Act 2005
MCI	Mild cognitive impairment
MDTs	Multidisciplinary teams
MMSE	Mini-Mental State Examination
NHS	National Health Service
NICE	National Institute for Health and Care Excellence
NSF	National Service Framework
PD	Parkinson's disease
PEG	Percutaneous endoscopic gastrostomy
PSA	Prostate-specific antigen
QoL	Quality of life
RCT	Randomized-controlled trial
RO	Reality orientation
SPECAL	Specialised Early Care for Alzheimer's
UCDS	Urban Community Dementia Care Services
UK	United Kingdom
UKCEN	United Kingdom Clinical Ethics Network
UN CRPD	United Nations Convention on the Rights of Persons with Disabilities
USA	United States of America
VBP	Values-based practice

Abbreviations

Introduction
Manifestos, Dementia, Values, and Rights

This is a book about dementia, but we are calling it a Manifesto because we want to change dementia care and the way dementia is understood by society in general.

We recognize that all the different health conditions that come under the umbrella term of dementia are real illnesses affecting millions of people worldwide, causing many people experiencing them or providing care genuine distress and debilitation. We fully acknowledge that as a progressive, terminal disease, without cure or evidence-based universally effective treatments, a dementia diagnosis may come as a devastating blow. We also recognize the importance of evidence-based approaches in trying to find causes, treatments, good care, and perhaps even cures for dementia.

But we have written this book because we also believe that dementia needs to be seen and understood as something much more than a collection of diseases requiring health interventions and other forms of support. Dementia is an issue about our common humanity – who we are, how we relate to each other, where we fit in society, and how society supports us when we experience difficulties. All forms of dementia have defied attempts to find a cure or truly effective treatments that stop the condition from advancing. Forty-seven and a half million people worldwide have some form of dementia, and because it is closely associated with ageing, this number will increase exponentially as people live longer and populations grow. Partly because of the fear and stigma that dementia invokes, having high-quality care and support is necessary but not sufficient to ensure those people can remain part of society and enjoy a good quality of life as much as possible, for as long as possible.

Our Manifesto builds on the work of others before us and tries to be inclusive of several different perspectives. We want to provide a kaleidoscopic yet clear view of what we believe to be important in the way people with dementia, their families, and their friends live in society and are supported. The dominant view of dementia is largely based upon a biomedical disease model. We do not reject this but stress the fundamental importance of also understanding it in terms of disability. People with dementia need care and treatment, but they also need to have their rights as citizens upheld, irrespective of the severity of the disease. We support the use of facts and evidence-based interventions where right and wrong are usually fairly clear. But much of this book focuses on *values*, on which we might disagree, where the language of right and wrong is usually not very helpful. Where a disease has no existing cure and the effectiveness of treatments is limited; where it has profound effects upon a person's ability to understand, communicate, remember, and many other basic human functions; where it is frequently described by phrases such as 'living death' (presumably making people with the disease the walking dead), under such conditions values must be addressed.

Values-based practice (VBP) is an approach that has been developed for health and social care practice to provide both a crucial counterpoise and partner to evidence-based practice (EBP). This book describes VBP and is the first book that applies it to dementia. But, call us foolhardy or brave, we wanted to do more than write a VBP guide for dementia. There are several reasons for doing this, but one that we wish to emphasize here is the importance of rights-based approaches for improving public services, including health and social care. A rights-based approach does not exclude or conflict with VBP, but VBP cannot afford to ignore rights. Rights are expressions of values but have solidity, because they are in the form of laws and legal conventions with processes enabling enforcement and challenge.

Structure of the Book

By realigning the values associated with dementia to focus on identity, agency, relationships, community, and rights, rather than a narrow focus on disease, dysfunction, despair, and ultimately, death, we hope this book can bring about change. Chapter 1 sets the scene, first by giving an overview of dementia and then by giving a summary of VBP. In Chapter 2, we describe how dementia really challenges VBP and present a growing emphasis on people's rights, including human rights, which we believe are of crucial importance. When we talk about values we are talking about action-guiding words for people. By realigning the values associated with dementia and incorporating a focus on rights, we are led to our Manifesto in Chapter 3. It's a very short and simple manifesto, but we believe that's what good manifestos should be, though we explain in the chapter some key themes that underpin it.

The book emphasizes that a focus on values, in partnership with evidence and rights, can really help develop and improve everyday practice in dementia care. By applying VBP, we believe some of the challenges and distress caused by dementia can be significantly mitigated. As well as being a Manifesto, the book is therefore also a guide to using a VBP approach in dementia care. Chapters 4–13 describe how VBP can be applied in practice. But we try not to lose sight of the Manifesto, so there are three layers to our book: people and dementia on top, supported by VBP beneath, and then underpinned by the Manifesto as a foundation.

Manifestos Again

So the book aims to change or influence practice as well as perceptions of dementia and provide guidance on how this can be achieved. Manifestos are often associated with change – perhaps the most famous manifesto, the Communist Manifesto written by Karl Marx and Friedrich Engels, was the source of considerable change, both good and bad. But manifestos can also describe ways of conserving and protecting what already exists. The Conservative Party in the UK produces manifestos before elections, and their ideology contains a strong emphasis on continuity and tradition rather than change. This is an apt reminder of how values may be immutable or deeply held by people, and, certainly, the task of dementia practitioners is not to change the core values, beliefs, or personality of a person with dementia or family carer they are working with. So this Manifesto also emphasizes continuity – of people, of relationships, of what makes us human. Finding ways of helping someone with dementia to preserve their identity, to continue to be able to communicate what's important to them, their likes and dislikes, their wishes, feelings, beliefs and values is an important task for dementia practitioners, as well as family carers. This can also be challenging, but there is plenty of evidence to indicate the importance of engaging and supporting the person, not just treating the dementia, even in the later stages of the illness. This is why we believe that it is crucial to understand dementia in terms of a social model of disability and in terms of rights, including human rights.

A word of caution: many of the challenges posed by dementia arise because the evidence and knowledge currently available about many aspects of the condition are still limited. The causation of most forms of dementia, finding more effective treatments than are currently available, and the subjective experience of the person with dementia as it becomes more severe over time are three of those challenges. Being aware of values and understanding them is useful in most situations but can be particularly important where evidence is more limited. VBP provides a process for doing this, but in some situations there may be no clear answers or simple solutions. Manifestos also have to take into account unknown or unpredictable factors since they are about the future – they rely partly on a willingness to believe, see, and do things differently. Tolerance of uncertainty, the unknown, and the unresolvable are useful adjuncts or skills to have (or cultivate) as ways of approaching those aspects of dementia involving limited knowledge or experience.

Calling a book a manifesto sets the bar very high in terms of ambition. We also think it's a new, positive, and stimulating way of thinking about dementia. VBP draws upon some philosophical thinking. Still, we concur with a quote from one of the authors of perhaps the most famous manifesto, Karl Marx, who wrote in his *Eleventh Thesis on Feuerbach*: 'The philosophers have only *interpreted* the world. The point however, is to *change* it' (the line also appears as an epitaph on his grave in Highgate Cemetery). This book describes the changes we aspire to in the world of dementia, but also some of the challenges – we hope that it will help readers work out how to address the challenges and change that world.

How This Book Was Written

We wrote this book as a joint endeavour but took responsibility for writing different chapters. We shared each chapter we wrote, sometimes on several occasions, and made suggestions and comments. It was a positive, constructive experience, and we both valued each other's expertise and experience enormously. The reader will notice differences in style between the chapters, but we decided that this was of potential benefit to the book and to the experience of reading it. Most importantly, we believe that our message is consistent, and how we apply the principles and practice of the Manifesto is the same throughout.

It may be useful for readers to understand our different backgrounds. Toby is an independent health and social care consultant working in the fields of adult mental health, dementia and disability, mental capacity, rights, and inclusion. He has worked in and managed frontline mental health services and has research, practice and service development, and policy expertise working at a national level in the UK, together with family experience of dementia. Julian is a consultant in old age psychiatry who has worked in multidisciplinary teams in various parts of the National Health Service in the UK looking after older people with a full array of mental health problems. He originally trained in general practice. He has been involved in a wide range of research but has a focus on philosophy and ethics in relation to ageing and dementia. His clinical and ethical interests are combined in his research on palliative care for people with dementia.

A Note on Terminology

In the book we generally use the term 'people' or 'a person with dementia'. On occasions, we use the term 'service user' or 'patient' where it makes the most sense in the context we are describing. We are aware that different people like some terms and dislike others, and we do not wish to offend or upset anyone. 'People' or 'person with dementia' is our preferred term because, first and foremost, this book is about people.

We often use the term 'carer' to denote family members or friends of a person with dementia who are also providing unpaid care and support to them. We fully recognize that family members and friends are people too and their relationships with a person with dementia they care for usually go far beyond just a caring role. 'Professionals' and 'practitioners' are the terms we use most to describe people in paid roles, though we appreciate there are staff and volunteers working in a wide variety of roles and settings doing invaluable jobs caring and supporting people with dementia, who might not use these terms to describe themselves. Wherever possible we try and be more specific about who a person is, but sometimes 'carer' and 'practitioner' are the terms that make the most sense.

Finally, we use the terms 'disease', 'illness', and (health) 'condition' fairly interchangeably to describe dementia (we also recognize that 'dementia' is itself an umbrella term). These terms can mean slightly different things, but our use of them is partly to differentiate them from describing dementia as a 'disability'. This is an important theme in the book, although we do not argue that they are mutually exclusive. However, we have always tried to use the term 'disability' in the context of a rights-based, social model of disability (which we shall describe in more detail later). 'Disability' in this sense refers to how wider society disadvantages, discriminates against, and excludes people with impairments, such as those caused by dementia. 'Impairments' describes the characteristics, features, or attributes within an individual which are long-term and may be the result of disease or injury, potentially causing pain and distress, but may also be deemed by society to be the grounds for excluding or rejecting the individual.

Manifestos, Dementia, and Values-Based Practice

Topics covered in this chapter
- We shall present an overview of dementia and values-based practice (VBP).
- We highlight key challenges that dementia poses that makes VBP relevant to our understanding of good dementia care.
- Dementia is described, along with its challenges.
- We consider VBP, its key components, good process, and its relation to evidence-based practice (EBP).

Take-away message for practice

The complexity of dementia sets challenges for VBP; but VBP establishes a good process by which to approach the complexities of dementia.

Introduction

A manifesto, according to the Oxford English Dictionary, is 'a public declaration of policy and aims, especially one issued before an election by a political party or candidate'. Perhaps the most famous manifesto, the Communist Manifesto, was central to the Russian Revolution and other revolutions across the world in the twentieth century. The intentions of this book are more modest – we are not declaring the formation of a new political party focused on dementia or demanding the overthrow of a government in order to change policy on dementia. But by having a manifesto as part of this book, we are calling for a mini-revolution in mainstream thinking, views, policy, practice, and lived experience regarding dementia. This mini-revolution involves a focus on *values* and *values-based practice* (VBP) to improve dementia care and the lives of people with dementia more generally. But we also believe that recent developments in policy and practice affecting dementia and the application of VBP to dementia care create challenges that require the manifesto to include other important factors such as rights, the complex interaction between dementia and values, and how we relate to each other as people to ensure the manifesto is relevant and meaningful. In turn, these factors provide new perspectives and insights regarding VBP. In other words, the application of VBP to dementia gives us new ways to think about dementia but also gives us new ways to consider VBP and, more widely, issues of our common humanity. This occurs, in particular, because of the salience of rights, personhood, and a notion of community we are calling *polis* when considering dementia.

This book describes the relevance of VBP to dementia and dementia care. The manifesto – set out in Chapter 3 – forms an integral part of the book and informs much of the thinking throughout. But we also show how the main process of VBP can be applied to dementia care generally. In order to do this, we start in this chapter by giving an overview of dementia and VBP and identify some of the key challenges that dementia poses which make VBP so relevant. In the following chapter, we discuss in more detail factors such as rights and the interaction between dementia and values that both challenge and enhance VBP. This then sets the scene for us to present the manifesto in Chapter 3 before describing the process of VBP in subsequent chapters; but we shall keep the principles established in the manifesto in mind throughout the book.

Dementia

Dementia is an umbrella term for a range of different conditions that cause damage to the brain. This damage affects a person's memory, thinking, communication, and ability to carry out everyday tasks. Dementia is usually a progressive, terminal condition and in many countries is now the leading cause of death. In 2015, in England and Wales, 61,000 people died of dementia – 11.6 per cent of all recorded deaths (Office of National Statistics, 2017).

Many conditions come under the umbrella of dementia. Alzheimer's disease is the most common (affecting around 50–75 per cent of people with a dementia diagnosis), but others include vascular dementia, Lewy body dementia, and frontotemporal degeneration.[1] There are some variations of symptoms across the different types of dementia (memory loss, though closely associated with Alzheimer's disease, is not the main symptom in some other forms of dementia). Research indicates that the most common risk factors for developing dementia (apart from ageing) include diabetes, hypertension, smoking, and low educational attainment at school (the latter is believed to be associated with having less cognitive protective capacity).

It is estimated there are 850,000 people living with dementia in the UK (Prince et al., 2014) and over 46 million people worldwide living with dementia. The risk of developing dementia increases with age; it affects one person in 14 over the age of 65 but one in six people aged over 80. As an 'ageing society', with more people living longer, it is estimated that there will be over a million people in the UK living with dementia by 2025. Ageing populations are a global phenomenon; the change is seen in national demographics the world over. Although diagnosis rates for dementia are improving, it is estimated that in high-income countries only 20–50 per cent of people with dementia are recognized and documented in primary care; and in low- to middle-income countries this figure could be as low as 10 per cent (Alzheimer's Disease International, 2011, p. 7). Yet in most forms of dementia a number of years elapse between the emergence of symptoms, the need for intensive or full-time care, and death.

---

[1] For further details and facts about the different types of dementia, a useful starting point might be Hughes (2011a).

There is no cure for dementia,[2] and the evidence base for treatments which delay the progress of dementia is still limited. It remains vital that researchers continue to look for possible treatments. There are some treatments, services, and supports that can help people living with dementia to have a reasonable quality of life. However, for the foreseeable future countries across the world are faced with the immediate challenge of caring for growing numbers of people with dementia with only limited interventions that ameliorate the symptoms, and none that reverse the underlying conditions that make up the dementias.

Key Challenges of Dementia

Although each person's experience with dementia is unique, people living with dementia, their families, professionals, and other staff who care for them face some common key challenges that are of particular relevance to this book:

- Dementia is a health condition, but the current limited evidence for effective health interventions means that there must be an ongoing focus on good care and support for people with dementia and their carers without the prospect of recovery.
- The mainstream perception and narrative around dementia are underpinned by a very negative set of values. 'Living death', 'apocalypse of the self', 'decreation', and the 'dementia tsunami' are typical of the words and phrases used in public and by the media. We do not deny that dementia can be extremely distressing for the person diagnosed with the condition and their family and friends, as well as challenging for practitioners. But perceptions of dementia that focus on a calamitous loss of self and agency, reducing the person to a passive and incapable victim/recipient of help, ignore, prevent, or bury personhood, including a person's values, beliefs, desires, biography, identity, and agency. At worst, the person becomes 'value-less' – not having values or being of value – which has serious ramifications for their safety and for the priority given to good quality dementia services. The person is seen to be totally subsumed by their dementia.
- As dementia progresses and becomes more challenging, care and support usually have to become more and more intensive, and it is usually harder for the person to express their needs and what they are experiencing. At its most

---

[2] The book uses the term 'dementia' as shorthand to denote the range of conditions which give rise to it. Elsewhere JCH (Hughes, 2011b, 2013) has argued that the term 'dementia' is problematic and should be abandoned, but the political saliency of 'dementia' is such that this does not seem likely to occur for some while. Still, in the *Diagnostic and Statistical Manual of Mental Disorders* (DSM) version 5, the dementias are now referred to as 'major neurocognitive disorders'. It is also worth noting that before 2004, the term for dementia in Japan was *chihō*. *Chihō* is a compound word: *chi* means foolish and stupid, and *hō* means foolish and absent-minded. When paired, both characters have connotations that can be interpreted as insulting and stigmatizing. In 2004, the term was officially changed as part of a public campaign to raise public awareness about dementia. The new name for dementia, '*ninchishō*', was selected. '*Ninchishō*' means 'recognition disease'.

severe, a person with dementia may lose all ability to communicate, be physically immobile, be incontinent, and be unable to perform simple personal tasks such as feeding or dressing themselves. They may also experience other long-term, severe health conditions and impairments associated with later life.

- As well as changes in a person's memory, cognition, and behaviour, dementia can manifest itself in unexpected or seemingly inexplicable changes in a person's beliefs and values.

- The changes described here may be accompanied by the person becoming more distressed and can result in carers, professionals, and other staff being confused or disagreeing about how best to respond. However, dementia alone does not automatically result in deterioration in a person's quality of life.

- The evidence base for some pharmacological treatments, psychological treatments, and a wide range of psychosocial, family, and environmental interventions that mitigate the negative effects of these changes is limited. As well as interventions being ineffective, they can sometimes be positively unhelpful and wasteful of resources.

- Disagreement and confusion, combined with the pressure on resources and time, which many dementia services currently experience, can result in poor decision making, conflict involving professionals, other staff, the person with dementia, and carers.

Apart from the difficulties caused by dementia to individuals, the cost of care for people with dementia is immense. It is estimated that dementia costs the UK £26.3 billion a year in terms of costs to health and social care services, the individual, and their carers (Prince et al., 2014). In residential care and nursing homes in the UK it is estimated that between 58 and 90 per cent of residents have dementia (2014). At least 25 per cent of UK hospital beds are occupied by a person with dementia (though dementia is not usually the primary reason for admission), and people with dementia tend to stay in hospital for longer than people without dementia. The longer a person with dementia stays in hospital, the worse the effect on both their dementia and physical health, making discharge more difficult and often resulting in the person being unable to return home and having to go into residential care instead (Alzheimer Society, 2009). In the UK, one-third of people with dementia live in residential care or nursing homes. Decisions about moving into a care home, especially from hospital, can be very distressing for individuals and their families, and may be the source of disagreement and conflict between professionals (Poole et al., 2014).

Dementia therefore represents one of society's most challenging health conditions, for individuals affected by it, dementia care practitioners, service providers, policy makers, and society at large. Both the condition itself and decisions about the most appropriate care for a person with dementia can cause confusion, misunderstandings, differing points of view, and conflict. This can be the source of further distress and poor use of resources. There is a limited range of really effective interventions and a limited evidence base to support many interventions. Dementia poses a fundamental challenge to mainstream biopsychosocial approaches to understanding disease and assessment, treatment and care. All diseases have a wider social component, inasmuch as they have an impact on family and wider society, but dementia contains a unique combination of factors which suggest searching questions about who we are, our place in the world, and about societal responses to challenges posed by incurable, non-reversible health conditions, and disabilities. This, in combination with a variety of views about the nature of dementia (as a biological disease, as a psychosocial construct, as a manifestation of normal ageing, as a failing, or as a highly stigmatized condition), means that decisions about a person's care frequently revolve around values and, where there are disagreements, around differences in values.

Dementia and Humanity

There is, however, a more positive way to regard dementia. This is not to deny or downplay how terrible the condition can sometimes be, but it is to emphasize something important about the humanity of people with dementia. In later chapters, we shall discuss the work of Tom Kitwood, who coined the notion of person-centred dementia care and talked about how the psychosocial environment can either encourage well-being or ill-being (Kitwood, 1997). In other words, the way people react to and treat people with dementia can either make them better or worse. Kitwood spoke of a 'malignant social psychology' surrounding people with dementia. Sabat (2001) has also spoken of 'malignant positioning', by which people living with dementia are made to feel incompetent, disabled (in a pejorative sense), useless, and so on. But both of these authors argue that things need not be so negative and suggest how agency, identity, well-being, enjoyment, contentment, and the like might be maintained by more positive attitudes. The Nuffield Council on Bioethics (2009) encouraged the thought that it is possible to focus on moment-to-moment experiences of pleasure and enjoyment to enhance the well-being of people living with dementia. This aim seems worth pursuing. The vision of living well with dementia is worth striving for, and it is more likely to be realized if what the person living with dementia values is placed front and centre. This focus also reminds us of our common humanity; how we would wish to be supported and cared for if we had the condition should encourage us to reflect on how we support and care for people living with dementia. And it also suggests that while a disease model may sometimes be necessary, it is insufficient in many situations to provide satisfactory responses.

Values-Based Practice

This manifesto applies VBP to dementia care. But what is VBP?

The first book in this series, *Essential Values-Based Practice* (Fulford et al., 2012), describes the key processes and skills of VBP, with the aim of helping clinicians acquire and develop them. At its heart VBP helps to address differing opinions on the best course of action to take, which can occur in consultations, meetings, and other encounters between people using services (including carers) and professionals (as well as other staff). These may arise, for example, where the behaviour of the person with dementia is challenging (e.g. agitation or aggression) and when clearly the person's values (even if they are entirely clear) are not congruent with what others are valuing. Similarly, a proposed move for someone with dementia into a care home may give rise to conflicts of values, especially where the person is resistant to the move (Greener et al., 2012). The disagreement may arise between the person with dementia and practitioners, between practitioners and families, between family members and the person with dementia, within families, between practitioners of the same profession or different professions, between some practitioners (but not all) and some family members, and so on.

If not addressed, disagreements and differences can lead to mutual distrust, dissatisfaction, ongoing conflict or disengagement, and poorer health outcomes. In some extreme situations, disagreements might even involve litigation.

VBP can also be used in situations where, even if there isn't a disagreement or conflict, it is useful to show that there is agreement *because* of shared values. It's a way of alerting those involved to the *possibility* of different views. It's a way to test decisions and to make people think harder or be more aware about the values guiding people's actions. Examples would be difficult decisions around the use of anti-psychotic medication despite their increased risks in people with vascular dementia, or decisions about whether or not to respond truthfully to a person with dementia who persistently asks the whereabouts of a deceased loved one in the knowledge that this will cause the person distress. Such decisions involve competing sets of values. When these decisions or situations are discussed by practitioners with families (and, if possible, with the person with dementia), it may turn out there is complete agreement about the best course of action to take, but it's still important to be alert to the possibility that someone may disagree. So VBP is important and useful even in the absence of disagreement and conflict.

It is also worth making the point that as knowledge about health conditions has advanced, together with improvements in health care and medical practice, factors to take into account and options for care and treatment have multiplied too. Many people living with dementia and their carers have also become more aware of their conditions and possible treatments. More choices, and more people involved in decision making, mean more values come into play. As one of the judges from the UK's Supreme Court commented in relation to the 2015 Montgomery Judgment on patient consent:

> Most decisions about medical care are not simple yes/no answers. There are choices to be made, arguments for and against each of the options to be considered.
>
> (Montgomery Judgment, 2015, paragraph 110)

VBP and Evidence-Based Practice

VBP can be seen as the other side of the coin or partner to *evidence-based practice* (EBP). EBP is an approach which encourages and helps practitioners to evaluate evidence, often from multiple sources, in order to ascertain the best base of evidence upon which to justify care and treatment decisions. Disagreements can, of course, occur even where there are two competing interventions, such as different types of medication, both supported by a robust evidence base. But there are often clear and agreed guidance notes, procedures, or hierarchies of interventions. EBP is an approach that is widely recognized, understood, and applied when making decisions about health and care interventions. Practitioners are likely to be trained in EBP, or at least be aware of it, and are usually cognizant of guidelines from professional and statutory bodies indicating the most appropriate interventions to use based upon the strengths of evidence supporting their efficacy. Where disagreements are much more likely to occur is in situations involving *differences in values* among those involved, where issues *other than factual evidence* inform people's views, opinions, choices, and decisions about the best course of action to take.

Typically, differences in values occur where there is only a limited evidence base for what works, or no evidence base at all, or where a service user rejects an evidence-based intervention for other reasons. It is perhaps no coincidence that VBP's origins were in psychiatry where:

- the evidence base for many health care interventions has been more limited or not as robust in providing cures or effective treatments compared with interventions for most physical disorders;
- there has been less concordance among many service users about the benefits of those interventions compared to their side effects;
- there have been difficulties in simply getting agreement and consent from service users who may be very distressed, cognitively impaired, or resistant to the intervention; and
- wider societal values quite explicitly come into play which include the use of coercion, perceived as necessary for protection or public safety, but sometimes experienced as oppression and social control.

We will often come back to these issues, and they are explored more thoroughly in relation to VBP and psychiatry (excluding dementia) in a workbook for mental health practitioners, *Whose Values?* (Woodbridge and Fulford, 2004).

Although VBP's origins may lie in psychiatry, there is now a growing body of literature on VBP, including the Cambridge University Press series of which this book forms part, and it is now being considered and applied in surgical care, commissioning, and interprofessional collaborative practice. There is also the Collaborating Centre for Values-Based Practice in Health and Social Care at St Catherine's College, The University of Oxford.[3]

Key Components of VBP

While VBP partly draws upon philosophical thought, as well as evidence and observations from practice, the key components of VBP can be described in fairly straightforward ways:

- *'Values' can be defined in many different ways and come from many different sources*. Definitions may include specific principles like respect for autonomy, beneficence, non-maleficence, dignity, non-discrimination, and being person-centred; but also more widely, values are at work when we talk about beliefs, morals, ethics, the ways staff and organizations should behave as described in codes of conduct and organizational policies, government policies, legislation, and the views on dementia expressed in the media and wider society. Values may be embedded and expressed in families, communities, social groups, and society as a whole. Most people's values will be derived from a range of different sources.

Reflection Point

If you have a few minutes to spare, try jotting down the answers to the following questions. Perhaps do it with one or two close colleagues and compare your answers.

What would be your important values? Could you list them, and how might your list differ from those of your colleagues? From where do your values derive?

---

[3] For more information see http://valuesbasedpractice.org/ – accessed 17 January 2017.

Personal values will be particularly important for service users or patients and carers; professional, organizational, statutory, and legal requirements will be particularly important for practitioners. Figure 1.1 illustrates how the sources of values overlap.

- *VBP advocates an inclusive approach to values,* recognizing they can be found in a whole range of situations and that everyone has them, although individuals may define them differently. People living with dementia and carers using services are not bound by professional or organizational values but by their own personal values, which may be based on a whole range of factors, including life experience; social, cultural, or political beliefs; religious conviction; and sometime idiosyncratic views of the world. Ask any group of people for their definition of values, and there will almost certainly be a real diversity in their answers – but also commonalities and a lot of mutual respect for other people's definitions, even where there are differences. VBP describes values as being like an extended family – there may at times be differences but they are still related!

- However we define values, we all have them. *Values guide our decisions and actions.* Practitioners working in dementia care have to be aware of their professional and organizational values (and sometimes their personal values) but also the values of others to help understand what a person with dementia is experiencing and to work well in partnership with carers and other practitioners. People with dementia and carers are likely to focus on their own personal values. The effects of dementia mean that the values guiding decisions or actions may not be clearly expressed. But, actually, none of us day to day is particularly good at defining the values that guide our actions. Often we just do things and do not realize, unless forced to, that what we have done has been driven by some particular value or other.

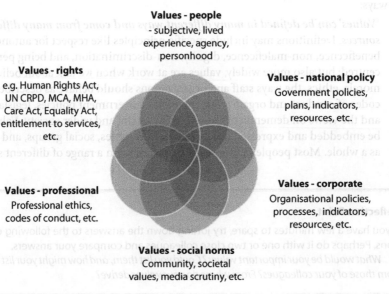

Figure 1.1 Different sources of values

Abbreviations: UN CRPD = United Nations Convention on the Rights of Persons with Disabilities; MCA = Mental Capacity Act; MHA = Mental Health Act.

- The *centrality of the patient/service user and their values* is fundamental. Practitioners should always use as a starting point the values of the person with dementia, but it is not the only point and will not necessarily determine the decisions and actions that need to be taken. Centrality does not mean totality, and the values of the practitioner, other staff involved in the person's care, and carers must also be considered.
- Values are everywhere and *there may be differences in values*, especially in dementia care, because there can be less agreement about why a person is behaving in a particular way or is distressed and how to respond than in physical health care. Important values to a practitioner may not be important to a person with dementia or their carer. Health care values can differ from social care values, and the values of different professional disciplines may also differ. Although there may be a prevailing consensus about a disease model for understanding and responding to dementia, this still leaves plenty of scope for practitioners to emphasize different values associated with the different components of the model in specific situations. And values beyond that model may also be relevant.
- *Shared values or a consensus about values* tends to occur where there is a common experience, view, or agreement about the facts and evidence relating to a specific situation. A simple example of this is to consider the differences between a 'good apple' and 'good art' (see the Reflection Point below).

Reflection Point

Here's another exercise you can do with colleagues when you have a few spare minutes.

How would you or your colleagues describe a 'good apple'? How would you or they describe 'good art'? Where is there most agreement and most disagreement about what makes an apple or art 'good'?

Note that this is a point about values too. We value certain things about apples that makes us call them 'good'; we value certain things about art that make us call it 'good'. There are also likely to be a lot more common words describing good apples than there are for good art!

Similarly, where there is limited evidence and a range of different views about what constitutes 'good care' for people with dementia, it is less likely there will be shared values or a consensus, compared with what constitutes 'good care' for people with diabetes, where there is much clearer evidence and agreement for the interventions that work. (It is interesting and important to notice, however, that even in the case of physical illnesses, like diabetes, there is still room for a divergence of values, especially at the margins of, say, mild type 2 (older-onset) diabetes: some value the benefits of medication, but some would wish to highlight the benefits of diet and lifestyle changes. Also, the values of some diabetics, such as teenagers with diabetes, might be very different from the values of others, such as their parents.) In this sense, facts and evidence are often value-laden. As in the case of 'good' apples, values are often shared or align with each other; but equally they can be at odds and divergent. As with diabetes, so, too, with dementia – research may generate evidence and facts about 'good' treatments. But even facts may be in conflict with each other, for example, effective treatments also having unpleasant side effects, so a 'good' treatment may also be experienced as a 'bad' treatment. And, as we shall discuss, even where there is almost universal consensus about the facts, such as around time, place, or identity, in dementia values can still throw up issues that challenge these facts.

- There can be **differences between explicit and implicit values**. Explicit values are those in which a person says they believe, such as a nurse talking about professional codes of conduct. But implicit values are ones which are not stated, or ones that a person may not even be fully conscious of, yet which influence their words and actions. For example, professionals may only loosely observe organizational policies because of pressure of time or resources (even if they explicitly state that such policies are valued); or they might subscribe to the values associated with a particular model of care over other models (e.g. a psychological model over a more biological or social model); or they might inadvertently apply personal values such as strong religious convictions or ageist assumptions when providing care. VBP research provides examples of this (Colombo et al., 2003; Mental Health Foundation, 2009). What we say about a situation and what we actually do about it may differ – this can be a cause of confusion and conflict if the difference is not acknowledged and, if necessary, discussed. Even if it is acknowledged and discussed, it may still be a source of disagreement, but at least people are being open and honest about the values that are guiding their actions.

- Being able to understand and work with the values that exist in situations involving dementia care is an essential part of VBP – **working in partnership** with others is essential. But using *facts and evidence* to understand what is happening and what to do when working with a person with dementia is an important part of VBP as well. In some situations, as in the case of effective treatments for dementia, facts and evidence may be weak or limited. But in these situations that is not a reason for dismissing whatever evidence exists and substituting EBP with VBP; the available evidence should still be considered on its merits in partnership with VBP where decisions clearly involve values as well. Working with facts **and** values is an essential part of VBP – it is crucial to be able to keep both in view and see both fields together, as illustrated in Figure 1.2.

- VBP does not generally say which are the 'right' or 'wrong' values because this often creates conflict (though we come back to this point later). Asserting that 'my values are right and yours are wrong' doesn't take into account all the preceding points about the ubiquitous, yet diverse, nature and prevalence of values. Instead, VBP aims to support *balanced decision making of shared values* (the main *point* of VBP), based upon *mutual respect for differences of values* (the main *premise* of VBP) within a given situation. VBP is therefore especially helpful where there is a disagreement or clash of values involving a person with dementia, carers, and practitioners.

- At a practice level, VBP translates these components into support for balanced decision making through *ten key elements of 'good process'*. VBP focuses on process, not outcome, because if the process for discussing and deciding on a course of action is one where all the different values are 'in play' – as well as evidence – and can be heard, respected, and considered, then the chances of a positive outcome are greatly increased and the risk of unhelpful conflict reduced. The ten key elements are divided into the following:

· four areas of clinical or practice skills;
· two aspects of professional relationships;
· three links with EBP; and
· basing partnership on what is referred to as '*dissensus*' as well as consensus.

'Dissensus' is used in this context not to mean disagreement but simply to mean, 'agreeing to disagree' about differences in values. Crucially, dissensus also means agreeing that all values *remain in play* and can continue to be referred to and that different values can be followed, depending upon how the situation develops.

The ten elements do not form a process that has to be followed sequentially, but are the key ingredients that need to be in the VBP 'pot' (added in no particular order) to make for a good stew (i.e. a good outcome)!

Clinical/Practice Skills

These are practitioner skills that are fundamental for any encounter with service users or patients, carers, and other practitioners in order to identify and work with the values (both positive and negative) that are present.

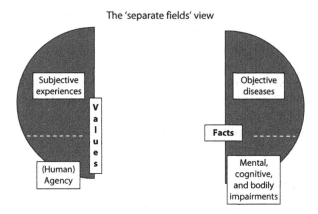

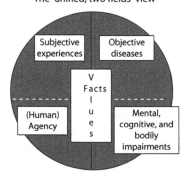

Figure 1.2 The 'separate fields' view and the 'unified, two fields' view

- **Awareness:** of the values present in any given situation. Paying attention to language is one way of raising awareness of values.
- **Reasoning:** thinking through the issues and consequences of the values involved when making decisions and taking action.
- **Knowledge:** understanding the values, and facts, relevant to the specific situation.
- **Communication:** using good communication skills to come to a balanced decision and resolving differences or conflict where there is values diversity.

Professional Relationships

Encounters between practitioners and service users are two-way interactions, at least, and often involve many more people, all of whom will have values. Practitioners need to be able to engage positively in these relationships and with these values.

- **Person-centred practice:** the first (but not the only) source of information on values in any given situation is the perspective of the person with dementia.
- **Multidisciplinary:** making positive use of the values diversity within teams, across disciplines, and with other services and agencies.

Links with Evidence-Based Practice

Focusing on VBP does not mean ignoring facts that are supported by EBP. Practitioners need to 'think facts; think values' (more on this in Chapter 8).

- **The 'two feet' principle:** all decisions are based upon consideration of values and facts or evidence.
- **The 'squeaky wheel' principle:** we only notice values when there is a problem.
- **Science and values:** advances in scientific knowledge create choices in care and treatment, which generate diversity of values. Science does not close down the possibilities for values diversity but often seems to open up practice (and society) to greater values diversity.

A Basis in Partnership

Partnership involves decisions being taken together by the person with dementia, carers, and the providers of care. Consensus is aimed at, but it is accepted that there may be differences of opinion (*dissensus*). In the absence of consensus about values in a specific situation, this should not mean having to decide whose values are 'right' and whose are 'wrong'. Keeping all values 'in play' is an important part of VBP.

Conclusion

This book draws upon all of these key components of VBP. However, to make it of practical use and benefit, it is structured around the ten key elements of VBP's 'good process' for balanced decision making within a framework of shared values and mutual respect for differences of values. The manifesto also builds upon the key components of VBP. But as we have already said, recent developments in policy and practice affecting dementia and the application of VBP to dementia care create challenges that mean the manifesto and VBP need to take into account other factors as well. The next chapter outlines these developments and challenges.

References

Alzheimer Society. (2009). *Counting the Cost.* London: Alzheimer's Society.

Alzheimer's Disease International. (2011). *World Alzheimer Report 2011: The Benefits of Early Diagnosis and Intervention.* London: Alzheimer's Disease International.

Colombo, A., Bendelow, G., Fulford, B., and Williams, S. (2003). Evaluating the influence of implicit models of mental disorder on processes of shared decision making within community-based multi-disciplinary teams. *Social Science and Medicine* 56, 1557–1570.

Fulford, K. W. M. (Bill), Peile, E., and Carroll, H. (2012). *Essential Values-Based Practice: Clinical Stories Linking Science with People.* Cambridge, UK: Cambridge University Press.

Greener, H., Poole, M., Emmett, C., et al. (2012). Value judgements and conceptual tensions: Decision-making in relation to hospital discharge for people with dementia. *Clinical Ethics* 7, 166–174.

Hughes, J. C. (2011a). *Alzheimer's and Other Dementias: The Facts.* Oxford: Oxford University Press.

(2011b). *Thinking Through Dementia.* Oxford: Oxford University Press.

(2013). Dementia is dead, long live ageing: Philosophy and practice in connection with "dementia". In K. W. M. Fulford, M. Davies, R. G. T. Gipps, et al., eds., *Oxford Handbook of Philosophy and Psychiatry.* Oxford: Oxford University Press, pp. 835–850.

Kitwood, T. (1997). *Dementia Reconsidered: The Person Comes First.* Buckingham: Open University Press.

Mental Health Foundation. (2009). *Model Values? Race, Values and Models in Mental Health.* London: Mental Health Foundation. Available at: www .mentalhealth.org.uk/sites/default/files/ model_values.pdf (last accessed on 9th October 2018)

Montgomery Judgment. (2015). *Judgement. Montgomery (Appellant) v. Lanarkshire Health Board (Respondent) (Scotland).* Issued by the UK Supreme Court in April 2015, [2015] UKSC 11.

Nuffield Council on Bioethics. (2009). *Dementia: Ethical Issues.* London: Nuffield Council on Bioethics. Available at: http:// nuffieldbioethics.org/project/dementia (last accessed 11 December 2017).

Office of National Statistics. (2017). *Deaths Registered in England and Wales (series DR): 2016.* London: Office of National Statistics. Available at: www.ons.gov .uk/peoplepopulationandcommunity/ birthsdeathsandmarriages/ deaths/bulletins/ deathsregistrationsummarytables/2016 (last accessed on 9th October 2018)

Poole, M., Bond, J., Emmett, C., et al. (2014). Going home? An ethnographic study of assessment of capacity and best interests in people with dementia being discharged from hospital. *BMC Geriatrics*, 14, 56.

Prince, M., Knapp, M., Guerchet, M., et al. (2014). *Dementia UK Update.* London: Alzheimer's Society. Available at: www .alzheimers.org.uk/sites/default/files/ migrate/downloads/dementia_uk_update .pdf (last accessed on 9th November 2018).

Sabat, S. R. (2001). *The Experience of Alzheimer's Disease: Life Through a Tangled Veil.* Oxford: Blackwell.

Woodbridge, K. and Fulford, K. W. M. (2004). *Whose Values?* London: The Sainsbury Centre for Mental Health.

Chapter

Enhancing Values-Based Practice and Developing a Dementia Manifesto

2

Topics covered in this chapter
- We highlight the challenges of dementia and the suitability of VBP to meet those challenges, even if this means expanding its scope, for instance, to include a more overt recognition of the place of rights.
- We consider the notion of 'right' and 'wrong' values.
- There are implications for VBP from scarce resources and from the weight of legislation and policy.
- Rights protect and empower people; rights may also serve to protect the values that are required for good practice in dementia care, and rights themselves reflect values.
- To the good process of VBP, therefore, we commend a rights-based approach.

Take-away message for practice
Right and wrong are always determined from some perspective or other. VBP encourages us to take a broad view of values and to understand their diversity. VBP needs to work with a rights-based approach.

Values-based practice (VBP) is a comprehensive and positive approach to difficulties that frequently arise in the provision of health and social care at the frontline when working with service users and carers. It acknowledges the importance of evidence-based practice (EBP) while also ensuring there is a focus on values, especially where facts and evidence are more limited in guiding choices and decisions. But for several reasons both dementia and policy frameworks for delivering health and social care more widely have, in recent years, created fresh challenges for implementing VBP in practice. These challenges are crucial in both enhancing VBP for dementia care and informing our Manifesto. When its key components are pushed to the limit, VBP might instead be described as 'VBP plus' or 'enriched VBP'. Dementia care today certainly points towards these enhanced versions of VBP. This chapter outlines these key challenges and explains how they enhance VBP and help inform our Manifesto.

Two Challenges of Dementia

Some of the practical challenges posed by dementia to VBP have already been described briefly in Chapter 1, and we come back to these throughout the book, showing how VBP can still provide a valid and practical approach to addressing them. But let's consider two key issues which put additional pressure on VBP.

Changing Values; Unknown Values

As the condition progresses, most forms of dementia can have profound effects on the person in terms of memory, communication, and understanding of self, place, and others around. For example, a person with dementia

a. May no longer recognize close family and friends and form new, sometimes intimate, relationships with strangers;
b. May believe they are a younger version of themselves, so that the past becomes the present ('time shifting');
c. May reject long-held beliefs, convictions, and rules of behaviour and act quite differently, sometimes exhibiting aggressive or disinhibited behaviour.

In other words, the values they held as being important before developing dementia – what guides their actions – may change quite dramatically. Sometimes it is possible to work out the reason for these challenges (e.g. by knowing a person's life story), but sometimes it may be a mystery as to why these changes occur or why the values underpinning them also seemingly change. And unlike all other major health conditions, the progression of dementia makes it harder and harder for the person to articulate reasons for these changes, and for others to understand. Although carers are invaluable sources of information about the person with dementia, this information may relate primarily to the pre-morbid values of the person. The carer may be equally bewildered and distressed by these changes. Sometimes, inadvertently, the carers' values are expressed instead of, or as if they were, the values of the person with dementia.

One can immediately see how much of a challenge these situations pose to several components of VBP and elements of its 'good process'. There are certainly a lot of values in play in these situations, but discerning what they are, and being able to communicate with the person with dementia about them, becomes highly problematic. Whether values are implicit or explicit, they may still be inexplicable. The four clinical/practice skills (discussed at the end of Chapter 1) are all made much more difficult by these developments. Person-centred practice is challenged fundamentally, facts and evidence are often of limited help, and 'squeaky wheel' situations become endemic.

Yet, as we hope to show, VBP can provide some solutions in these situations. And it is worth holding on to the final element of VBP's good process, partnership involving 'dissensus', as an important way of approaching and trying to develop solutions. Accepting that dissensus may be the only practical way forward in supporting or caring for the person, finding new, sometimes unusual (even uncomfortable) ways of working in partnership with the person and others – and in this context applying the other elements of the VBP process – may provide some answers.

'Right' and 'Wrong' Values

Following on from the difficulty of knowing or understanding the values of a person living with dementia, a second fundamental challenge posed by dementia relates to VBP's aim of moving away from 'right' and 'wrong' values because of the conflict this can create.

The key premise in VBP of mutual respect for differences of values underpins the importance of not asserting one set of values as being the 'right' ones (e.g. the importance of treating someone with an evidence-based intervention) over what might appear to be the 'wrong' ones (e.g. patient autonomy, where someone with capacity is refusing the intervention for idiosyncratic reasons). Conflict, disengagement, and poorer health outcomes in the longer term may well result when the views (based on divergent values) of those involved do not coincide. A person's values may appear to be idiosyncratic, unwise, or based upon beliefs without factual evidence, but practitioners regarding them, and certainly designating them, as 'wrong' or 'bad' is likely to damage the therapeutic relationship and violates the element in VBP of service-user centrality.

VBP acknowledges that there are some exceptions, most notably when values are discriminatory in some sense (i.e. intentionally exclude other values). Racism is an obvious example – it's intolerant of diversity and therefore violates the premise of mutual respect for different values. But dementia shines a torch in more complex areas where there are other distinctions between right and wrong, good and bad, that pose different kinds of challenges. Let's consider Mr Patel.

Mr Patel

Mr Patel is a 90-year-old Hindu man who was born in India and came to the UK in the 1970s, having lived in Uganda for a time before being expelled by President Idi Amin. He has always lived in a predominantly Hindu area. He was diagnosed with Alzheimer's disease three years ago, although he has consistently refused to acknowledge the diagnosis despite presenting with clear symptoms. His GP tells him that everyone gets a bit confused and forgetful as they grow old so there's nothing to worry about. Mr Patel's wife died two years ago, and the rest of his family have little contact with him apart from one adult daughter and a grown-up granddaughter who look after him in his home.

Recently Mr Patel had a fall and was admitted to hospital via the emergency department with a hip fracture. Mr Patel is now recovering after surgery on a general medical ward. According to his daughter, Mr Patel is much more confused than he was before being admitted to hospital. He frequently shouts racist abuse at other patients and staff working on the ward who are African-Caribbean or whom he believes to be Muslim, saying 'don't touch me', and keeps trying to leave, saying he doesn't want to be 'locked up in here'. He is particularly hostile to a female consultant, who is Muslim and wears a headscarf, and towards a male African-Caribbean social worker who is trying to arrange his discharge, and has attempted to hit both of them. Although he used to speak English, now he speaks mainly in Hindi. Since being in hospital Mr Patel has also rejected his usual diet and keeps on asking for beef burgers. His daughter insists he should not be given these, as his religion forbids it, but Mr Patel gets angry when his request is refused.

The daughter and granddaughter know that Mr Patel lost most of his possessions when he was expelled from Uganda. They also recently found out that he served in the Indian Army and was involved in the war with Pakistan in the late 1940s and was briefly held captive by Pakistani soldiers. They say that Mr Patel was never hostile or aggressive towards Muslims or African-Caribbean people in the past and was always very polite when he had contact with them (including when they were health care staff). However, they said in private he had expressed mistrust of Muslims and African-Caribbean people and didn't like his family having contact with them.

The example of Mr Patel illustrates five different dimensions to the discussion around 'right' and 'wrong' values:

a. *Even 'wrong' values may have understandable reasons.* It appears that Mr Patel's values involve prejudice, if not racism, towards African-Caribbean people and Muslims. However, his experience of living in and fighting for India, shortly after the partition with Pakistan, and his expulsion from Uganda may provide the explanations for this, even if they are not justifications. However, it is unclear why Mr Patel is so keen suddenly to eat beef burgers, though it is always possible that witnessing the advertising campaigns of famous fast-food outlets may have tempted him in ways he was previously able to resist.

b. *Values are different from actions.* Mr Patel has probably held these values most of his life, but until recently has not publicly acted upon them. Until recently, therefore, even if Mr Patel's (inner) values are deemed to be wrong (or even 'bad'), his actions in public were 'right'. Even so, expressing values (especially racist values) within the family might have had a big impact on them: for good (they may have overtly rejected them) or for ill (they may have covertly agreed with and absorbed them). And acting upon these values by verbally abusing or hitting people is clearly wrong. But is Mr Patel's wish to eat beef burgers and disobey the values of his religion of the same magnitude in terms of being wrong? Should the distress it may cause his daughter be equivalent to the distress caused by his apparent racism? Thus, should the staff resist his racism but comply with his desire for beef or vice versa? Should they resist or go along with both? On what grounds would we wish to discount religious values but uphold social values or vice versa?

c. *Dementia may disinhibit the expression of 'wrong' values and actions.* The effect of Mr Patel's Alzheimer's disease seems to be a significant factor in how he is now expressing his values and his actions. But being in hospital also seems to be a trigger. His values and actions seem to be influenced by being in an unfamiliar environment where he feels trapped and with some people whom he feels threatened by, resulting in him being fearful and hostile. Although his values *and* actions may be 'wrong', they are perhaps based upon Mr Patel trying to make sense of the situation. He may have 'time shifted' in order to do this, believing himself to be in the army again or in Uganda (as also indicated, perhaps, by his reversion to speaking in Hindi). Likewise, his desire for beef burgers may be based upon a reaction to the advertising he has witnessed. With the loss of short-term memory but retention of long-term memory and 'emotional memory' (as opposed to factual memory), unfamiliar situations can be reinterpreted and re-experienced as replicating or re-creating emotionally important events from the past.

d. *Dementia can accentuate the differences between right and wrong.* All the signs indicate Mr Patel believes he is a young man again and being held captive by Pakistani (Muslim) soldiers, harassed by black Ugandans, but also at liberty to eat beef. His understanding of his age and being in hospital is incorrect; this incorrect understanding is bringing out the 'wrong' values resulting in 'bad' behaviour. The distinction is so clear, based upon the facts of his situation, that surely one can say that that Mr Patel's values are 'wrong' and that the hospital is a 'good' place for him to be. But it is precisely situations like this where keeping the focus away from right and wrong is so important. These expressions of 'wrong' values may be difficult for everyone, but it is most difficult for Mr Patel because, on account of his cognitive impairment, he will find it hardest to understand what is happening, to appreciate the distress he is causing, and to modify his behaviour. Although Mr Patel may fluctuate between his 'dementia-orientated reality'[1] and the factual reality of his situation, it is only likely to confuse and distress him more by telling him that his beliefs and values about the situation are wrong (let alone 'bad') when he is experiencing the different reality. However, this in turn potentially creates difficulties for others about right and wrong. If Mr Patel is not told the truth, isn't that wrong, especially if a (well-meaning) lie is told to him? Dementia care sometimes creates situations where truth-telling causes more distress ('good' values leading to a 'bad' outcome), but the alternative (not telling the truth) causes moral, ethical, professional, and practical problems ('bad' values perhaps leading to 'good' outcomes). We shall come back to truth-telling in Chapter 5.

e. **Dementia can undermine facts, based on shared values.** Despite the fact of being diagnosed with Alzheimer's disease, Mr Patel refuses to acknowledge he has the condition. This may be because of the dementia, but may also be because he consciously or unconsciously does not want to accept that he has dementia. It is not uncommon for people to deny they have serious, long-term conditions, and denial is protective in some ways. But denial can also be revealing of the person's values concerning identity, health, illness, and possibly shame or stigma. But as Mr Patel's dementia gets more severe, this clearly poses greater problems in terms of engaging him with health and social care. Mr Patel's general practitioner (GP) is colluding with this, perhaps for benign reasons with respect to Mr Patel's wellbeing, perhaps because he doesn't really know much about dementia, or perhaps because of an implicit belief that very little can be done for Mr Patel ('therapeutic nihilism'), or perhaps because he doesn't really care. Whatever the reason, the GP is rejecting some facts and being guided (rightly or wrongly) by particular values.

Similarly, values associated with the belief in our own senses and cognition about identity and place are nearly always implicit – based on our self-knowledge, knowledge of others, and where we are in terms of location – and are normally consistent with the values of those around us. This means there is usually no debate about the facts concerning who or where we are. For Mr Patel, however, this is not the case. His beliefs about identity, time, and place may make perfect sense to him but are fundamentally different to his family and the staff caring for him. Situations where a person with dementia believes a deceased parent or partner is still alive are also examples of discordant facts. Even facts, therefore, become unsteady and sources of possible dispute or distress. Loss of factual memory but retention of emotional memory (and what we might call 'values memory') make VBP's person-centred practice and its 'good process' much more challenging. These

---

[1] 'Dementia-orientated reality' (DOR) should not be confused with 'reality orientation' (RO) for people with dementia. Although both are practice tools for people with dementia experiencing different realities, the former accepts and works with that reality, whereas the latter attempts to 'reorientate' the person back to the factual reality apparent to everyone else. For more information on DOR see Caiazza and James (2015). For more information on RO see Spector et al. (2000). A more general discussion of the issues of different realities experienced by people with dementia can be found in Williamson and Kirtley (2016).

challenges are not insurmountable – this book aims to explain how they can be overcome – but it does require extra mental and ethical dexterity!

Values expressed by a person with dementia may appear to practitioners and carers to be very wrong, or even bad, and certainly not reflecting the factual reality of a person's situation. Because of their own values, staff and carers can therefore find it hard to know how to react.

In fact, this situation also occurs with patients who do not have cognitive impairment: some may just (for whatever understandable or non-understandable reasons) seem to be 'bad' people who do and say 'bad' things. Staff must still respond in a professional and non-judgemental manner. But in this case they can, in a sense, be open about their professional response: they can, for example, state that racist language is not tolerated in the hospital but can meanwhile continue to give professional care. In the case of Mr Patel, they are more conflicted because they know that he would not formerly have said such things, that it is 'the dementia talking', and that telling him the hospital's policy will do no good, so they are not inclined to lecture him. Moreover, they know they should regard him positively, but they are upset by what he says and does.

The situation with Mr Patel also reminds us about the need to continue to place the person with dementia 'front and centre' as we described in Chapter 1, challenging though this may be. Unnecessarily negative or judgemental responses by practitioners indicate a loss of sight of our common humanity as well as of the effects of dementia. Caring for people who are unwell can be difficult at times, when a person is expressing unpleasant views and behaving in difficult ways, but they are still persons with rights and in need of support, not rejection or condemnation.

Although dementia challenges VBP's perspective on 'right' and 'wrong' values, far from negating this perspective, it shows how important it is still to try and apply it. Dementia can result in right and wrong appearing to be or mean something very different to the person living with dementia than it does to others and can make it very difficult for the person to understand or change. Chapter 4 returns to the issue of right and wrong and describes some of the philosophical and ethical approaches to this issue.

Two Wider Challenges

In addition to the specific challenges posed by dementia to VBP, many countries over the last few years have seen very significant changes in policy and legislation governing health and social care, which in turn have had a significant impact on dementia practice. These create pressures on key components of VBP.

The Value of Resources

Since the financial crisis of 2008, many countries have significantly reduced or stopped increasing public expenditure on health and social care services. For example, spending on health care in the UK between 2009–10 and 2014–15 grew at only 1.1 per cent per year, the slowest growth rate since 1955–56. In a similar period spending on adult social care fell by 6.4 per cent, at the same time as the population aged 65 and above grew by 15.6 per cent (Luchinskaya et al., 2017). Yet this has coincided with a growing increase in demand for those services as populations age and life expectancy increases. At the frontline, practitioners frequently find themselves with growing caseloads but often with fewer colleagues and limited or non-existent services that they can work in partnership with to provide care and support. *'Values-based practice is all very well but I simply don't have the time or resources to implement it'* is a sentiment that is often expressed. Furthermore, countries like the UK offer free, universal health care, but social care is both financially (means) tested and restricted by rigid eligibility criteria, resulting in the majority of people with dementia having to meet the costs of their social care themselves ('self-funders') or being primarily supported by family and friends.

VBP has no direct answers for the practical difficulties caused by the pressure of too little time and too few resources. VBP is also clearly practice-focused and non-political and so does not address issues of funding for services. Nevertheless, decisions to increase or reduce funding for services are informed by values, albeit ideological ones, and VBP needs to acknowledge this. At a practice level, implementing VBP needs to take into account issues of staff time, resources, availability of services, and funding mechanisms to ensure that it remains relevant and useful. This means that in dementia care VBP needs to be as simple as possible to implement guiding actions without being turned into cumbersome systems or procedures, additional meetings, targets, or mountains of paperwork.

But pressure of time and resources can also lead to hasty or impulsive decision making where, for example, a practitioner believes they are right and ignores the views and values of others, resulting in an inappropriate course of action being taken and poorer outcomes. Indeed, the lack of time makes VBP all the more important: it is more important to get things right (or as right as they can be) the first time, to establish the right sorts of relationships with service users or patients and their carers at the outset, to understand the different values at play from the beginning. We believe that the ten key pointers of 'good process' can easily be used without falling into the trap of becoming over-systemized, but still enabling a pause for collective thought about what is important to all concerned. This can actually reduce time wasted in intractable debates about the best course of action, inappropriate use of scant resources because of poor decision making, and poorer outcomes, which often occur when there isn't a proper focus on values.

Legislation and Policy

Closely connected with the issue of resources is the issue of legislation and policy. Laws contain values that a society has agreed upon and that have been enacted through a political process. Laws are based upon shared values concerning what is wrong (e.g. murder), when the state has the right to intervene in someone's life, the entitlements citizens have to certain services and opportunities to participate in community life, and other societal rules and norms.

Policies may be more ideological in tone, reflecting the views of the government of the day, and therefore certainly contain values and require organizations and individuals to act in particular ways. Most policies do not come with the full weight of law behind them (though may use elements of legislation to help with implementation), but place statutory requirements on organizations and individuals, and implementation is carefully monitored.

In a sentiment similar to the one expressed about resources, practitioners may well say, 'Values-based practice is all very well, but the most important thing is that my practice is lawful and I follow policies and my professional and organizational guidelines'. Over the last 25 years that sentiment has been further complicated in many countries by the increase in policies and legislative frameworks affecting people with dementia.

In 1995, a person with dementia in England could be detained and treated in hospital under the Mental Health Act of 1983 if they met certain specific criteria, and they also had statutory rights to social care services, public housing, a state pension, and welfare benefits. There was no human rights legislation, disability rights or mental capacity legislation, and no national policy for dementia.

In addition to numerous legislative changes to the health and welfare systems in general, Table 2.1 describes pieces of legislation, international conventions, and policies that have come about since 1995 relevant to a person living with dementia in England in 2017.

Table 2.1 Legislation, Conventions, and Policies Affecting Dementia Care in England

Legislation and conventions	Brief description (and key values)
Human Rights Act 1998 (UK-wide) – applies the European Convention on Human Rights (ECHR) to the UK	General protections, drawn from the ECHR, e.g. • Article 2 – right to life • Article 3 – prohibition of torture, inhumane or degrading treatment • Article 5 – right to liberty and security • Article 8 – right to respect for private and family life • Article 10 – freedom of expression
Mental Capacity Act 2005 – MCA (applies to England and Wales; similar, equivalent legislation in Scotland and Northern Ireland)	• Protects the right to make decisions and advance planning • Clear processes and safeguards where someone lacks capacity to make decisions (best-interests decisions) • Covers consent and other decisions regarding assessment, treatment, detention, and care, including end-of-life decisions and research
Mental Health Act 1983 (amended in 2007; applies to England and Wales; similar, equivalent legislation in Scotland and Northern Ireland)	• Allows compulsory detention and treatment for mental disorders without consent
United Nations Convention on the Rights of Persons with Disabilities (UN CRPD) – ratified by the UK in 2009 (UK-wide) Note: The CRPD is a UN treaty that the UK has agreed to comply with, but it does not form part of UK law	Describes positive rights for people with disabilities, including: • Respect for dignity, autonomy, participation, inclusion, and differences • Equal recognition before the law • Access to and provision of accommodation, support, health services, reablement, work, justice, and community and civic life
Equality Act 2010 – includes disability rights (UK-wide)	Prohibits discrimination on the grounds of disability and age, for example
Care Act 2014 – comprehensive social care legislation (and equivalent legislation in Wales, Scotland, and Northern Ireland)	Describes statutory rights to social care and support services (including carers)
Policy documents	
Living Well – National Dementia Strategy for England (Department of Health, 2009) (Wales, Scotland, and Northern Ireland all developed their own dementia strategies)	Seventeen objectives including raising awareness about dementia, diagnosis, treatment, care, housing, service commissioning, workforce development, and support for carers
The Prime Minister's Challenge on Dementia (Department of Health, 2012) (England only)	Three main objectives: improved diagnosis, health, and social care for people with dementia; increased dementia research; and the development of better awareness through 'dementia-friendly communities'
The Prime Minister's Challenge on Dementia 2020 (Department of Health, 2015) (England only)	Built upon the objectives in the 2012 'Challenge' with an additional objective on risk reduction for dementia

NB! In the MCA, "best interests" is felt not to be compliant with the CRPD in this respect.

An increase in the number of legal frameworks and national dementia policies has occurred internationally since the 1990s. Since 2007, over 80 countries have ratified the UN CRPD, which requires national policies and laws to be compliant with the rights of people with disabilities (disability is defined to include mental impairments caused by conditions such as dementia). A recent survey of legislation covering capacity to consent to treatment in Europe found that 28 countries had either passed or updated legal frameworks since 1990 and 28 new pieces of legislation had been passed since the year 2000 (Alzheimer Europe, 2016).

In terms of policies, France can lay claim to being the first major country to introduce a national dementia strategy in 2001. There are now at least 35 countries around the world which have national dementia strategies or plans (Alzheimer's Disease International Dementia Plans and Alzheimer's Europe National Dementia Strategies). These plans often incorporate indicators of progress in their implementation. For example, in England over 30 indicators were developed as part of a statutory public health profile for dementia, showing data relating to the prevalence, prevention, and care of people with dementia. (This Public Health England Dementia Profile may be found at https://fingertips.phe.org .uk/profile-group/mental-health/profile/dementia).

What does this increase in legalization and policy mean for values and VBP in dementia care? It certainly signifies an increase in the range of values that practitioners have to take into account. Whereas in the early 1990s, VBP might have focused primarily on values of the service user and carer and the professional and clinical values of practitioners, now there is a much greater array of legal, organizational, and policy values that affect dementia care. Values (often changing) associated with the reconfiguration of services, collecting data, reporting on outcomes, and having services and practice scrutinized are everyday experiences for many practitioners. But values associated with rights expressed through legal frameworks is an area that we believe requires a particular focus in relation to VBP and dementia.

The Challenge of Rights

We recognize that responding to corporate and policy values creates additional pressure on practitioners and the implementation of VBP, but we are particularly interested in values expressed through legislation, as these affect VBP in very significant ways. First, laws are the most (democratically) forceful way of expressing societal values (although they may still generate some dissent) and contain the most severe sanctions if they are violated. Second, they increase and reinforce the rights of service users and carers and a sense of entitlement (albeit this is sometimes not an accurate reading of the law). At the same time, legislation can be used by practitioners to make decisions or take actions (including denying services) which have neither been requested by nor meet the wishes of service users or carers. And finally, although legislation may offer legal protections for practitioners, it may also be the source of anxiety or fear: for service users and carers, a loss of liberty, being stigmatized, or refused help if subjected to the law; for practitioners, very serious consequences can ensue violations of the rights of a service user, including the possibility of a professional no longer being able to practise, or even facing criminal charges.

Thus, rights are a theme we return to frequently in this book, because they are such an important form of values, but also because, generally speaking, they appear fixed and immutable and do draw a clear distinction between right and wrong. Service users, carers, and practitioners may see rights in terms of good and bad – certainly in situations where a service user or carer is being abused or wilfully neglected, but also where they are being applied correctly, as in, for example, compulsory treatment. Table 2.1 provides a snapshot of the vast array of values in the form of rights that can apply to people with dementia. In the UK, these range from rights involving consent, assessment, and access to health and social services (e.g. MCA, Care Act) through to broader citizenship rights and protections (e.g. Equality Act, UN CRPD). Using the same examples of legislation, rights may also relate to an individual, defined in their relation to a service (e.g. a person potentially needing to be detained in hospital or entitled to social care) or to people who are members of an ethnic minority, are disabled, have a different sexual orientation, or because of age or gender, for example, are at risk of being unfairly discriminated against.

As well as becoming more ubiquitous, rights operate much more like facts despite appearing to be more like values. In situations where legal frameworks apply, the values expressed in law are likely to have more weight than other values, such as the preferences of a service user or carer. So this could make the premise of VBP – mutual respect for differences of values – problematic if practitioners believe the law must be applied. In turn, this could skew the 'good process' of VBP towards what is lawful and upset the point of VBP: balanced decision making within a framework of shared values. Similarly, a service user may assert their right to refuse a health or care intervention and use the law to ensure this is respected, even if it appears unwise or potentially harmful to the eyes of practitioners and carers.

It is important, however, not to lose sight of the values that underpin legislation. Mental health and mental capacity legislation have usually been based on a sometimes uneasy combination of values involving respect for individual autonomy, protection of the individual from harm, and public safety, and are compatible with the disease model. On the other hand, equalities legislation and the UN CRPD are underpinned by a 'social model of disability'. The key difference between this model and the disease model is that the former focuses on societal changes (e.g. public attitudes and behaviours, physical environments, provision of support, etc.) to enable people with disabilities (and the impairments caused by dementia mean that it can be legally defined as a disability) to live as full and equal citizens. The social model of disability developed from a social justice movement made up of people with a range of disabilities and their supporters, who saw institutional and charitable responses to people with disabilities as patronizing, discriminatory, and oppressive. Disability in this sense describes political, social, economic, and cultural processes of excluding and disadvantaging a person with impairments, such as those caused by dementia, and can be seen as akin to racism or sexism. On this basis it is incumbent upon society to change the environments, practices, and behaviours which exclude rather than trying to 'fix' the individual and the condition that gives rise to their impairments. There are different iterations of the social model and ongoing debates between them, which place more or less emphasis on the subjective experience of disability, especially for people with cognitive and mental impairments. The exclusion of people with impairments described by the social model of disability includes a lack of public concern or investment in researching and providing interventions that mitigate the impairments so it does not reject per se the importance of care and support for individuals.

There is a further set of values that underpin the CRPD which connect with the social model of disability, or what some call the 'human rights model of disability' (Alzheimer Europe, 2017). These are values of active inclusion and enablement for people with disabilities, rather than values concerned with prohibitions on discrimination, equalities, and freedoms. Several articles in the CRPD refer to states taking appropriate steps and measures to ensure that people with disabilities have access to education, employment, and income, and can participate in the political, cultural, and recreational life of their communities. In this sense, rights not only provide protection for people with disabilities but also positively emphasize the need to enable people to participate in community life as citizens, equal to those people without disabilities.

Historically, dementia has not figured significantly in debates about disability, whether academic, policy, or practice related. Yet the cognitive impairments caused by dementia and the fact that social models of disability are all firmly located in a 'human rights–based approach' to disability make them both relevant and applicable to people with dementia (Mental Health Foundation, 2015; Alzheimer Europe, 2017). Shakespeare, a sociologist who argues in favour of disability rights, goes further in debates with colleagues, where he argues that a human rights approach in dementia should be founded on the basis of relationships and partnership, as well as the lived experience of the person living with dementia (Shakespeare et al., 2017) and,

> taking dementia seriously means reconfiguring our approaches to disability as a whole. The condition of dementia challenges the disability community to remember how impairments can impact daily living, and how emotionality is important. It also reminds us how humans can communicate and connect without language, and that we are more than our memories. (2017, p. 9)

It is worth noting that the increased focus on rights has partly come from people with dementia, which focuses both on rights involving consent, care, treatment, and so on, but also wider disability and citizenship rights. In Scotland, people with dementia were actively involved in producing a charter of rights for people with dementia and their carers (Alzheimer's Scotland, 2009). Several publications explore the rights of people with dementia (Mental Health Foundation, 2015; Hare, 2016), including a guide to human rights written by an international organization of people with dementia: the Dementia Alliance International (Dementia Alliance International, 2016). In 2017, submissions based upon the views of people with dementia in the UK were made to the UN committee responsible for reviewing compliance with the CRPD (Alzheimer's Society, 2017; Dementia Policy Think Tank, DEEP Network, Innovations in Dementia, 2017). A clear call was made in 2018 for human rights and social justice in an editorial column in the *Journal of Dementia Care* written by two people with dementia (Hullah & Dunne, 2018).

It is important, therefore, not only to understand legislation and rights in order to practise lawfully but also to be able to identify and understand the values that those frameworks contain. The five principles in the MCA and the 'wellbeing' principle in the Care Act provide examples of where these values are clearly stated in the law (Box 2.1).

In relation to the human rights–based approach, various tools are available to help operationalize this approach in policy and practice which clearly expresses values. These include the 'PANEL' principles and 'FREDA' (Box 2.2).

VBP in dementia care is pushed further, not only by the growing legal framework, but also by quite radical values that inform some elements of that framework. Although VBP has never ignored legal frameworks, the need for practitioners to be 'rights compliant' creates real pressure on upholding its key premise, process, and point.

Box 2.1 Examples of Principles from UK Legislation

Mental Capacity Act 2005 (covers England and Wales)

- Every person (adult) has the right to make his or her own decisions, including adults with particular medical conditions or disabilities, and must be assumed to have the capacity to do so, unless it is proved otherwise.
- A person must be given all practicable help and support to make a decision for themselves before anyone decides the person lacks capacity to make the decision.
- People have the right to make decisions that others disagree with or that appear unwise or eccentric, and it cannot be assumed they lack capacity for this reason.
- Any decision made or action taken on behalf of someone who lacks mental capacity to make a decision must be done in their best interests.
- Any decision made or action taken on behalf of someone who lacks mental capacity to make a decision must take into account whether it could be done in a manner that would interfere less with the person's rights or freedom of action, providing it is still in their best interests.

Care Act 2014 (covers England only)

- Every local authority (public providers of social care) has a duty to promote an individual's wellbeing when carrying out a range of functions for adults with care and support needs and their carers.

Box 2.2 PANEL and FREDA Principles

PANEL Principles

Participation – people with disabilities can participate in decisions affecting their human rights

Accountability – there is monitoring of organizations' adherence to human rights affecting people with disabilities and taking remedial action where necessary

Non-discrimination and equality – all forms of discrimination and unfair treatment of people with disabilities are prohibited

Empowerment – people with disabilities are given the information and support necessary to enable them to participate in decision making and claim their rights

Legality – rights are recognized as legally enforceable entitlements by public authorities

(Adapted from the Scottish Human Rights Commission, 2009)

FREDA Principles

A human rights–based approach to health care (Curtice and Exworthy, 2010).

The following principles should be embedded in everyday professional practice in relation to patients:

Fairness

Respect

Equality

Dignity

Autonomy

A Rights-Based Approach as Partner to VBP?

Although VBP emphasizes the values of the patient or service user as being the starting place, it does not describe a sequence or hierarchy of values to be considered – this would contradict VBP's resistance to describing values as right or wrong and undermine the premise of mutual respect for differences of values. However, the challenges described earlier seem to point to a need to understand the differences *between* values, not just the values themselves in isolation. The nature and implications of values differ, as do the relationships between them. To paraphrase a famous adage, fittingly for a manifesto, but to use it more democratically, 'all values are different, but some are more different than others'!

The relative immutability and factual appearance of values reflected through rights are perhaps the clearest example of the extent of these differences and provide grounds for arguing that they require a slightly different approach. VBP is not an all-encompassing approach, but recognizes that there are other practice frameworks with which VBP works in partnership, such as EBP. We believe that a rights-based approach (or 'rights-based practice') is another vital partner to VBP, and has become more so as legal frameworks have proliferated. Just as the resources of VBP can be complemented by the resources from scientific research, so it can also be complemented by resources found in the law, making it more likely that the point of VBP – balanced decision making within a framework of shared values – can be achieved. The fact that some rights are based upon a disability model of dementia, rather than a disease model, adds new values to situations. This may make things more challenging, but it also enhances the application of VBP by introducing new ways of understanding and responding positively to the lived experience of dementia.

Of course, at times there will be tensions within a rights-based approach, and between it and VBP or EBP. The dynamic between promoting wellbeing, autonomy, and safeguarding and responding to dementia as a disease or disability clearly contains potential for conflict. But, as already indicated, VBP does not aim to describe the 'correct' outcomes – rather it aims to provide a process by which good, satisfactory, or acceptable outcomes can be achieved. Incorporating a rights-based approach as a partner into this process, recognizing it as a separate but important tool in the toolbox, is wholly in keeping with the principles of VBP.

However, it is important to retain the focus on partnership (tripartite in this case), not hierarchy. Despite the seeming weight and force of law, in many situations it may not be particularly relevant, nor be the source of values most in play. Personal convictions can be deeply held and difficult to shift, while areas of the law which are permissive (i.e. allow things to be done, such as advance planning), rather than prohibitive (banning things from being done), may be unnecessary or irrelevant (or sometimes overlooked). A high-profile incident reported in the media about poor dementia care can make social norms feel like very intimidating values to practitioners (i.e. values they cannot ignore).

Having an understanding of values being expressed through legal frameworks (or scientific evidence) and seeing these as partners to VBP may help clarify what 'differences in values' means in practice. One could say it's like the difference between stone and water – they are tangible physical substances made up of chemicals, but other than that they are totally unlike each other. Both have very different uses, and they can interact with each other in helpful and unhelpful ways. There's no point in arguing which is the more important or whether they are good or bad.

Clearly context and situation are crucial – sometimes it will be clear that legal frameworks apply, and sometimes it will be much more nuanced around the personal values of the person with dementia and his or her carers. VBP emphasizes the importance of being aware and knowledgeable of all the values in play in any given situation, but a conception of VBP working in partnership with other frameworks may help to provide a focus on those values which require the greatest attention.

To help identify the relative importance of values expressed through a rights-based approach in relation to VBP in a particular situation, questions such as the following may be useful to ask:

- How strongly held are the relevant values of the person living with dementia? Have these changed as a result of the dementia? Has the person expressed different values or acted contrary to these values in the past?
- Are there legal rights/legal frameworks which clearly apply in this situation?
- Is there a clear risk of violating someone's rights or acting unlawfully?
- Does a code of conduct or organizational policy give clear guidance on how (or how not) to act? Are there exceptions to this?
- Does scientific evidence provide helpful indicators of a good course of action?
- How strongly held are the values of the person's carer(s)?
- What aspects of a disease model or a disability model of dementia (or both) might be helpful for the person with dementia, carers, and other practitioners in this situation?

We have emphasized the importance of rights for a number of reasons, but it is worth remembering that some rights are specifically referred to as human rights. This is a good reminder that rights are more than just legal frameworks and should reflect shared values of our common humanity. Despite some ongoing debates about the application of human rights, there is a fairly common understanding concerning how they express fundamental values about how we should live together and treat each other, irrespective of our individual circumstances such as disability or illness. A rights-based approach used in partnership with VBP and EBP must always retain a focus on people supporting each other through our connectedness and interdependency. Perhaps more than most other health conditions, dementia is as much a social phenomenon as it is a medical phenomenon, affecting the lives and identities of everyone it touches, so it requires a response that draws upon a broad range of disciplines, knowledge, and person-centred approaches.

Conclusion

This chapter, along with the first, has introduced readers to dementia and given an outline of values-based practice. But this chapter has also identified ways in which dementia, developments in health and social care and disability politics push VBP to its limit and perhaps beyond. The issue of 'right and wrong' values and rights in the legal sense are two examples where questions are posed of VBP. An enhanced understanding and application of VBP can still provide ways of addressing seemingly intractable challenges. The rest of this book is structured around the ten key points for 'good process' in VBP as it applies to dementia, whilst taking account of the additional challenges in dementia care that have been described. In this sense, the book aims to be a guide for VBP in dementia care.

We believe, however, that the issues VBP raises for dementia and the particular challenges posed by dementia, along with the wider developments in health and social care and disability politics, merit something in addition to a guide, in fact, a Manifesto. This Manifesto draws upon VBP, together with the other challenges we have described, and speaks to dementia practice in the twenty-first century.

References

Alzheimer's Disease International Dementia Plans. www.alz.co.uk/dementia-plans [Last accessed 7 December 2017].

Alzheimer Europe. (2016). *Dementia in Europe Yearbook 2016. Decision Making and Legal Capacity in Dementia*. Luxembourg: Alzheimer Europe.

(2017). *Dementia as a Disability? Implications for Ethics, Policy and Practice. A Discussion Paper*. Luxembourg: Alzheimer's Europe.

Alzheimer's Europe National Dementia Strategies. www.alzheimer-europe.org/ Policy-in-Practice2/National-Dementia-Strategies [Last accessed 7 December 2017].

Alzheimer's Scotland. (2009). *Charter of Rights for People with Dementia and Their Carers in Scotland*. www.alzscot.org/ assets/0000/2678/Charter_of_Rights.pdf

Alzheimer's Society. (2017). *List of Issues in Relation to the Initial Report of the United Kingdom of Great Britain and Northern Ireland [In Relation to the CRPD]*. Via: www.alzheimers.org.uk/download/ downloads/id/3631/submission_to_ uncrpd_committee_on_dementia.pdf [Last accessed 11 December 2017].

Caiazza, R., and James, I. (2015). Re-defining the notion of the therapeutic lie: Person-centered lying. *Faculty of the Psychology of Older People (FPOP) Bulletin*. Leicester: The British Psychological Society.

Curtice, M. J., and Exworthy, T. (2010). FREDA: A human rights-based approach to healthcare. *The Psychiatrist* 34, 150–156.

Dementia Alliance International. (2016). The Human Rights of People Living with Dementia: From Rhetoric to Reality. Retrieved from: www .dementiaallianceinternational.org

Dementia Policy Think Tank, DEEP Network, Innovations in Dementia CIC. (2017). *Our Lived Experience: Current Evidence on*

Dementia Rights in the UK. An Alternative Report to The UNCRPD Committee. Via: http://dementiavoices.org.uk/ wp-content/uploads/2017/07/Our-Lived-Experience-270717_1.pdf [Last accessed 11 December 2017].

Hare, P. (2016). *Our Dementia, Our Rights*. The Dementia Policy Think Tank and Innovations in Dementia CIC.

Hullah, N., and Dunne, T. (2018). Rights are for all. *Journal of Dementia Care* 26(1): 3.

Luchinskaya, D., Simpson, P., and Stoye, G. (2017). *IFS Green Budget 2017*. London: Institute for Fiscal Studies.

Mental Health Foundation (MHF). (2015). *Dementia, Rights and the Social Model of Disability. Policy Discussion Paper*. London: Mental Health Foundation.

Public Health England Dementia Profile. http://fingertips.phe.org.uk/profile-group/ mental-health/profile/dementia [Last accessed 7 December 2017].

Scottish Human Rights Commission. (2009). *Human Rights in a Health Care Setting: Making It Work – An Evaluation of a Human Rights-Based Approach at The State Hospital*. Glasgow: SHRC, pp. 10–11.

Shakespeare, T., Zeilig, H., and Mittler, P. (2017). Rights in mind: Thinking differently about dementia and disability. *Dementia*, 0(0): 1–14. DOI: 10.1177/1471301217701506

Spector, A. E ., Orrell, M., Davies, S. P., and Woods, B. (2000). Reality orientation for dementia. *Cochrane Database of Systematic Reviews* Issue 3, Art. No.: CD001119. doi: 10.1002/14651858.CD001119.pub2.

Williamson, T., and Kirtley, A. (2016). *What Is Truth? An Inquiry about Truth, Lying, Different Realities and Beliefs in Dementia Care (Review of Evidence and Report)*. London: Mental Health Foundation.

Chapter 3

The Dementia Manifesto

Topics covered in this chapter
- We introduce the three principles of our Manifesto:
  - Dementia as humanity
  - Dementia as disease and disability
  - Dementia, values-based practice (VBP), and rights
- We discuss some metaphysical, ethical, and political notions which underpin the principles of the Manifesto and also discuss:
  - Personhood
  - Values
  - Rights
  - The *polis* (our definition of community)

Take-away message for practice

Our views about dementia reflect our views about humanity; people with dementia have rights; both disease and disability models are relevant to understanding dementia; VBP with attention to rights provides a means to safeguard the rights and humanity of people with dementia.

A manifesto is a public declaration; it's also a showing forth, making something manifest. Our aspiration in this book is to demonstrate facets of dementia which show something about the reality of living with dementia and indicate radical implications for dementia care and are fundamental to our ways of living together. These form the basis of our Manifesto and deserve to be publicly declared. We believe they can also encourage change or action in the way society thinks about dementia and responds to dementia and people affected by it.

The Manifesto is quite simple and consists of three key elements or principles:

- ***Dementia as humanity.*** Dementia is a unique touchstone for understanding disease and disability, self-identity, aspects of the human condition such as ageing and mortality, a person's place in society, and how we live together as people, families, and communities. Dementia therefore reflects key aspects of humanity. Appreciating both the expressed and implicit values of people living with dementia, those who provide support, care, and treatment for them, as well as how society values dementia, provides invaluable insights into who we are as people and how we relate to each other. At the same time, understanding and appreciating those same values, wherever possible, are essential to how we support people to live well with dementia, how we provide care and treatment for them, how we support those around them (both staff and family carers), and how we educate the wider society about dementia. Our perceptions, understanding, and practical responses must incorporate, and yet go beyond, a disease model of dementia.

- *Dementia as a disease and a disability.* In Chapter 2 we described the challenges that dementia, resource pressures, and the proliferation of legal frameworks pose to VBP. Two further issues, recurrent themes in this book that we have already alluded to, are also of fundamental importance to the Manifesto. They can be symbolized as a dyad in the way that dementia is experienced, conceptualized, and understood, as well as how society, policy makers, services, practitioners, and carers respond to people with dementia. They epitomize an apparent tension which our Manifesto seeks to address. One view is that dementia is a disease, akin to other diseases, like cancer, for example. This sees dementia in the context of a biomedical model that emphasizes interventions involving cure, treatments, and care for the individual. The second theme is the view that dementia is a disability. This emphasizes the social and political aspects of dementia and focuses on what wider society must do to adapt and accommodate people experiencing the impairments it gives rise to. We shall argue that both themes must be played and heard at the same time.

- *Dementia, VBP, and rights.* Values-based practice (VBP) provides an essential framework for providing support, care, and treatment to people with dementia and their families and friends. It is built upon an awareness and understanding of the values described in the 'Dementia as humanity' principle. Using VBP in partnership with evidence-based practice and an applied understanding of rights enables us both to use and move beyond a disease model of the condition and will significantly enhance both the quality of life and the quality of care for people living with dementia.

Our Manifesto's three principles suggest rather a grand scheme, because we wish to get to the roots of the problem with which we are confronted. The problem that faces us is that of dementia and how we deal with it. So note, it's not *people living with* dementia that are the problem. Part of the motivation for this Manifesto is the conviction that there is something wrong with the ways in which we understand and deal with dementia now. And although this does imply that most people living with dementia struggle in some sense or another, it implies more than this. It reflects the *fundamental* nature of our declaration, because it also implies something about how we live together today.

Dementia is a problem because of the challenges it poses. These are not unique to dementia, but dementia presents the challenges uniquely. It represents a challenge to our sense of mortality. It's a challenge to our sense of self or personhood. It's a challenge to our standing as autonomous agents capable of determining our lives through the decisions we make. It's a challenge to our sense of dignity. It's a challenge to our place in society, to the roles we play in our families, to our relationships and identities. It's a challenge to our humanity.

Perhaps for these reasons (and others), it's a challenge that many people say they cannot face: it's the condition that some people say they most fear. Moreover, it's a challenge that is increasing in its prevalence as the population worldwide ages. From this perspective it's seen as an economic, social, and political challenge. Its biological connections with ageing mean that it raises fundamental challenges for science that are both empirical and conceptual. How, for instance, do we mark out the space of normality when people at a relatively young age already carry the pathological hallmarks of the disease (Hughes et al., 2017)? It raises practical, clinical, and ethical challenges for health and social care systems all over the world. It raises social and legal challenges to do with care, treatment, and disability, where people living with dementia receive care in the community but also in institutions, sometimes under specific legal frameworks. There's the challenge of abuse – of people living with dementia by their carers or people employed to care for them, and of carers by those for whom they care. And yet despite all of this, we hear that you can 'live well' with dementia (Nuffield Council on Bioethics, 2009). A VBP approach supports practice that promotes the notion of 'living well with dementia', but this phrase contains values in its own right which we will come back to in later chapters.

Themes in Tension

First, there is the theme that dementia is a disease, akin to other conditions. The observable signs of dementia such as the atrophy of the brain arc incontrovertible and are supported by evidence about risk, cause, and possible treatments. This justifiably gives rise to research and biopsychosocial interventions aimed at preventing, halting, or reversing the illnesses that cause dementia. The stigma and ignorance that have surrounded dementia must be dispelled because they prevent dementia from being prioritized as a health condition that must be tackled by policy makers, researchers, and services. As with any other health condition, people with dementia, or those caring for someone with the diagnosis, have rights to health and social care to address their needs. In the same way that cancer is now talked about much more openly, treatments have improved, and survival rates increased, so, too, must the same happen for dementia. Yet thus far, successful treatments and interventions for dementia have proved elusive or remain limited in their effectiveness.

Second, the contrasting theme is that dementia is a disability, like motor neurone disease or multiple sclerosis. The impairments caused by dementia affecting cognition, communication, memory, behaviour, and motor skills are well evidenced. The single biggest risk factor for most forms of dementia is still the inevitability of the ageing process. For the foreseeable future dementia remains a progressive and terminal condition experienced by millions of people around the world, who will live with it for the rest of their lives. The lack of progress in finding effective and acceptable treatments for dementia requires that in the meantime society must uphold the rights of people with dementia: they live with a disability, but they are still full and equal citizens. People with physical disabilities, sensory impairments, and, to some extent, learning disabilities have challenged stigma and discrimination, partly because they have also challenged the biomedical framework that defined the condition. Yet this has not happened to the same extent for people with dementia; it is not commonly recognized as a disability, and despite its limitations, the biomedical disease model of dementia remains dominant, including among many people with dementia.

The tension between a biomedical disease model and a disability model is played out in debates, decisions about resources, information, service configuration, and day-to-day interactions with people with dementia and their families. Should these activities continue to focus on a disease model of dementia and biopsychosocial interventions, or a disability model which has a more explicit rights focus and seeks to make society more accommodating for people with dementia? This book shows how both models are underpinned by values in combination with facts and rights, so the answer to such a question has to incorporate both models and the values underpinning them but also challenge the premise of the question itself and simply say it is not an either/or situation.

Our contention is that the duality should not involve choosing one or the other. Both themes are relevant to individuals and families affected by dementia, practitioners, services, policy makers, communities, and society. Seeing dementia as disease can provide understanding and some amelioration of its effects in the here and now, and may generate solutions in the future, but still remains limited in what it offers to people currently affected by the condition. Viewing dementia as a disability has the potential to change current perceptions of dementia and people's lived experience of the condition by altering in a positive way how society responds to dementia, supported by legal frameworks requiring institutions and individuals to adapt, accommodate, and include people with dementia as citizens like anyone else. But a disability model should not be used as an excuse to reduce efforts to understand the biomedical aspects of dementia or to continue to seek effective interventions. The values underpinning one theme must not be used to deny or marginalize the values of the other.

Much of this book will reflect our concerns about persons, values, rights (disability rights and human rights), and the *polis* (as our way of defining community). But before we get to the level of thinking about persons, values, rights, and the *polis*, to understand our positive declarations, it's necessary to look at the fundamentals that motivate our thoughts. These will move from the metaphysical to the ethical and then to the political.

Metaphysics

The idea that we are going to talk about metaphysics will seem daunting to some. But we only mean that we wish to consider the nature of the background from which we approach the problems raised by dementia. To sound more metaphysical, we could speak of the nature of our *being in the world*. Here we wish to commend the human person perspective. In other words, we take it as read that people see the world (including dementia and everything to do with it) from the point of view of human beings. Moreover, we are all people for whom the world *means* something, not just in one way, but in many ways. We see things as being biological, psychological, social, spiritual, ethical, political, cultural, legal, geographical, and so on. Things we see in the world have these many different types of meaning. The point about the human person perspective is that it is not circumscribable (Hughes, 2011; pp. 241–49). It cannot be shut down. There are always multiple ways to see things. There is no limit to the ways in which things in the world might have significance for real people. And people with dementia are real people, too, even if they have cognitive impairments or communication difficulties which make it harder for them to express their perspectives. The world *means* something to them, but unlocking that meaning may be challenging.

Meaning and significance also convey a sense of values: they guide action and reflect what's important for individuals, families, communities, groups of common identity or experience, and societies.

What follows is that we approach dementia as a layered phenomenon: it's biological, psychological, social, spiritual, ethical, political, and so forth, and is saturated with values at virtually every layer. But it's not one of these things on Monday and a different thing on Tuesday. It's all of these things at once. Dementia is multilayered, multifaceted, multifarious, multidimensional, etc. In other words, individual people, including people with dementia, cannot be understood in one way only: we all have multiple ways in which we can be understood. So, too, a person living with dementia is a physical being, capable of being studied by biological scientific methods but is, at the same time, a cultural person potentially capable of having views on how things should be done under this or that circumstance. Our ways of *being in the world*, that is to say, are both factual and evaluative – and this is true of all of us. If people with dementia can be explained in terms of brain function and dysfunction, they are also 'valuers' (Jaworska, 1999): they have views on things, perspectives on the world, which will range from complex views on political matters to more straightforward views about what they like to eat. The facts about us are different, but so, too, are the things that have meaning and value for us. Although it may be vital to consider the values of others, the person living with dementia must remain at the centre of the conversation about their lives and their care, and their agency and personhood must be held in focus and supported.

The metaphysics, understanding the nature of our being, can take us into difficult waters. For there is a narrow conception of what it is to be a person which excludes people with dementia, because it suggests that we are essentially cognitive beings, defined as persons by our cognitive abilities and disabilities. Our stance, however, is that such a view is too restrictive (see Hughes 2011b for a fuller discussion). The human person perspective is from a situated or embedded position in the world where we are partly constituted by what surrounds us: physically, psychologically, socially, spiritually, morally, and so on. We are not disconnected from our surroundings, which play a real and sometimes critical role in defining us as persons. Our physicality, our embodiedness (the visible way we express our feelings and thoughts), is itself not just a factual matter. From the human person perspective, our bodies are also connected to the ways in which we understand the world. Our bodies convey our meaning as well as allow us to understand the world as meaningful. And where meaning appears, so, too, do values.

We ourselves, including our bodies, are also temporal. We exist in time: we have a past as well as a future. We have not come from nowhere, and where we are projects us into the future. Our histories help to define us and are therefore vital to an understanding of who we are. To some extent at least, it is our past that defines our present and throws us forward into the future. A shorter way to say this is to note that we are situated or embedded in our narratives, in our stories, which have a beginning, middle, and end. We can think of ourselves as narrative beings, in which case (again) understanding our histories, as well as our cultures and traditions, becomes vital as a means to understand who we are. All of this is as much the case for people living with dementia as it is for everyone else. To paraphrase Marx, writing in *The 18th Brumaire of Louis Bonaparte* (which was published in 1852), 'We all make history but not under the conditions of our own making'.[1]

This foray into the metaphysical, therefore, has shown the extent to which we are, by our nature, human beings for whom things have meaning in a multiple layered manner.

---

[1] The full quote (translated by Saul K. Padover from the German edition of 1869) is as follows: 'Men make their own history, but they do not make it just as they please: they do not make it under self-selected circumstances, but under circumstances existing already, given and transmitted from the past'. Available via: www.marxists.org/archive/marx/works/1852/18th-brumaire/ch01.htm (accessed 5 January 2018).

We, as human beings, can be described in factual terms – we are physical beings – but we are also valuers who see the world in an evaluative fashion. We are situated or embedded in multiple domains, which exist at one and the same time, so that our embodiedness links with our emotional and intellectual being too. And an understanding of us *as selves* requires an understanding of the nature of our narrative selves, of our histories, as well as of our interconnectedness (our relationships) with others and with the world.

Ethics

If the metaphysics implies that there are multiple ways in which we can be *our selves*, the ethical stance we adopt is underpinned by the idea that there is something *that it is* to be ourselves. Following the existentialists, we might speak of a 'true' self or of an authentic way to exist or be in the world. Whatever that might mean (and, of course, philosophers have debated and contested the notion of authenticity), it suggests that for each one of us there is a way – and perhaps a number of potential ways – for us to flourish, to be the sort of beings that we should be. Our use, therefore, of the notion of 'ethics' is deliberately intended to reflect the broad notion of ethics outlined by Aristotle (c. 384–c. 322 BC), who also wrote of metaphysics and politics (as well as of biology, logic, and many other things). We are certainly not speaking of a limited vision of ethics such as that epitomized by the (so-called) four principles of medical ethics (Beauchamp and Childress, 2001). Our notion of ethics would include such principles, as well as those from the field of person-centred care as espoused by Tom Kitwood (1997); it involves a broad view of social, psychological, biological, and spiritual realities and multifarious human phenomena.

It is not our intention to stipulate how people should behave generally (albeit we are saying things about how to behave with respect to people living with dementia) – we are not setting out a universal morality! – but we do want to say that certain behaviours will allow us to flourish and others will not. On the whole, being dishonest, bullying, ungracious, inconsiderate, unkind, unreliable, cruel, self-centred, greedy, unfaithful, obnoxious, and dictatorial are not good ways to be. 'On the whole', of course, because there may be individuals who have to be some of these things under certain circumstances or because such behaviours are deeply ingrained patterns inculcated from their earliest years over which they have, perhaps, had little opportunity to exert control. But, *on the whole*, such traits and dispositions neither create nor manifest human flourishing.

However, *on the whole*, the world is a better place when people can flourish by being compassionate, loving, honest, faithful, dependable, gracious, giving, kind, considerate, brave, concerned for others, just, helpful, true, joyful, trustworthy, and so forth. Thus, the virtues describe the dispositions required to live well. From ancient times they have epitomized the good life. Vices do the opposite: they describe how we should live if we wish to make life miserable for ourselves and for those around us. VBP is on the side of human flourishing. Even when confronted by behaviours that are challenging in people living with dementia, or similar behaviours in their carers, or even difficult behaviours from colleagues, the values-based practitioner will be prone to try to understand the behaviours in a way that is both helpful clinically (e.g. behaviours that challenge can be regarded as manifestations of unmet needs (cf. James and Jackman, 2017)) and ethically (e.g. because practitioners must place the person living with dementia centre stage whilst taking a balanced view of all the values in play).

People who live with dementia will also wish to live flourishing lives. Why would they not? Sometimes this is not possible. People who live in poverty, people living in the midst of war, people living in corrupt societies, people who experience exclusion and loneliness will all find it difficult to flourish. The ethical imperative to do something about poverty, war, and corruption, however, is a reflection of our desire that people should be able to flourish. We value free, open, caring societies in which people can participate in a transparent manner, where decisions are made with a view to helping the worse off no less than those able to do well. Even in such situations and societies where there is cruelty, corruption, and suffering, the smallest acts of compassion and kindness are valued even more because they provide a glimmer of hope and of the good life. So people living with dementia may find themselves in difficulties because of their conditions, but the ethical imperative is still to do something – anything – that will help. This may be as little as a kind word or a hand for reassurance. Small gestures can make a big difference.

We have put this in terms of flourishing and the virtues, where virtue ethics goes back to the time of Aristotle. There are, of course, alternative approaches to ethics. The philosopher Immanuel Kant (1724–1804) highlighted the golden rule – that we should only do to others as we would wish them to do to us and that we have a duty never to treat people merely as means, but rather as ends in themselves. The other major ethical theory, utilitarianism, summed up in the writings of John Stuart Mill (1806–1873), suggests that the ethical thing is to maximize pleasure or happiness. All three major ethical theories can be used to support our contention that, on the whole, the world will be a better place when people behave towards one another in ways that are courteous, kind, considerate, and so on. That there will be disputes between theorists as to which approach is best should not deter us from our main ethical claim: there are ways for us to be in the world that will make it a better place. And these ways of being can be described by words that sum up what we value: kindness, compassion, honesty, and so forth.

Incidentally, we are not for our purposes interested in which particular ethical theory a person might subscribe to; we prefer here simply to say that any theory of ethics that works will be one that describes and defends the things that we value as human beings. But not just anything, of course. Our stance is that human values, if they have an ethical basis, must be valued for their contribution to human flourishing, to the good way of being human described by the virtue words. Furthermore, human values are important or valued because of the duties we have towards one another as ends, not solely as means to an end. They must also be valued because we believe they help to make the world a better place by maximizing real human happiness, pleasure, wellbeing, or something else that we consider worthwhile. In short, human values reflect what we consider to be significant and meaningful. It is this that makes them ethical in the sense that their significance and meaning make them the sort of things we feel we ought to do insofar as we wish the world to be a better place. Of course, how people define what's worthwhile or things like 'happiness' can vary dramatically, so values will differ enormously and may come into conflict with each other. Working out what is significant and meaningful in practice will often therefore be contentious and messy, but it's the reality of the world we live in.

Nevertheless, it is still possible to argue, as we have done, that *from a practical point of view* values as such should be regarded as ethically neutral. VBP requires this. It is just that if we wish to seek an ethical basis for particular values, we should do so by looking at the significance and meaning by which they contribute to the world being a better place. Our contention is that in almost every case we shall find that a person's values do play this role. It also allows, however, that there may be some people – very few – who are genuine sociopaths, whose values (insofar as they are sociopathic) would never win the day, even if they had to be recognized as part of the process of VBP.

Thinking about ethics, therefore, as in the case of metaphysics points in the direction of human beings as valuers. Moreover, if you are to understand a person's values, you will also need to understand his or her history. We are again confronted by the importance of narrative. Narrative ethics indeed might be a sensible approach to the difficulties of ethical decision making in the face of human complexity. The complexity of our values emerges in the complexity of our narrative selves. The focus on values also points towards the inevitability of negotiating around our values in order to discover how we can best flourish. But the need for negotiation moves us from ethics to politics.

Politics

Ethical decisions at a communal level become political decisions. Politics is about ideas, but it is also about action. How we live together in communities is the stuff of politics. Politics is about the communal life of the *polis*: the Ancient Greek word for the city-state or political community.[2] There are ways for us to work things out, for instance, by a democratic process. Although we live in a democracy and regard it as the best process for allowing decisions to be made between conflicting parties, it is not our concern here to argue in favour of a particular system (nor to excuse the obvious deficiencies of democracy). Instead, we would wish to argue that the practices we adopt should enable people to flourish, enhance wellbeing, and allow our values to be supported but also contested and at times developed by the force of open argument. If this could happen under a benign dictator, then all very well. But, of course, benign dictators can become malign; a well-intentioned individual can become too removed from the multifarious needs and values of his or her contemporaries, and almost by definition, dictators are known for being the sole arbiter of how decisions are made, ignoring or suppressing the rights and views of others.

There would be an argument in favour of liberal institutions focused on the civil rights and entitlements of individuals, as well as an argument in favour of communitarianism (perhaps a type of collectivism), with its emphasis on the social aspects of life, from our identities to our relationships, from our real to our virtual institutions, to include our social and economic rights as well. But dementia forces both views on us: what is required is a liberal, individualistic, *and* communitarian (or collectivist) society. We should lose neither the civil and political rights of the individual nor the notion of the embeddedness of the individual in an inevitable mesh of interdependency and interconnectivity, themselves constitutive of personhood and the framework of collective rights which express this embeddedness.

The difficulty for any community of individuals will come when they disagree. When values are shared, the *polis* can work very well. The virtues or vices of any particular political system will become apparent when the system has to negotiate between competing values. Any decision in a state or community of any size and complexity, albeit one that on the whole encourages human flourishing, is likely to upset some of its members. It is quite possible for a *polis* to take a decision that favours the less well-off and the minority. Such a decision is likely to upset the interests of someone, such as the interests of a richer elite. However, it is when the *polis* takes decisions that leave someone disadvantaged,

---

[2] We have chosen to use the term *polis* as it denotes both the interconnectivity of individuals, families, social groups, etc., in a community but also the political parameters of a community (which could be a nation but also a city, local government area, etc.).

especially when the people concerned are already powerless, that the notion of rights tends to appear.

Political activity in its broadest sense produces rights. Rights are the antidote to political power. The government may wish to make a decision that seems correct, but at times these may override or come into conflict with people's entitlements and legal frameworks, including human rights; a rights-based approach which focuses on these is a means of establishing other values that need to be heard. Ethics is about flourishing individuals; politics is about the good life of the community. But rights emerge as a way to protect individuals in the face of the community's interests when these run counter to established legal frameworks. We discussed rights in the previous chapter, but it's worth reiterating that when we refer to rights, we mean both universal rights, that should benefit everyone whoever they are, such as human rights, and the rights of specific groups, such as disability rights. People are 'rights holders'. Some rights are limited or come with conditions, such as the rights to services one has as a citizen of a particular country. Other rights are absolute and without conditions for the rights holder, such as not being subject to inhumane or degrading treatment or punishment; but these clearly create conditions and responsibilities for 'duty bearers' – those people (such as healthcare professionals) who should respect, promote, and implement the rights of the people for whom they care. Rights under national laws, as well as international human rights, include both absolute and conditional rights, and having a way of understanding and applying them where relevant is crucial.

Within this broad context, it is almost inevitable that we should start to speak of the rights of people living with dementia. It would be, and historically it has been, easy for disadvantaged sections of society to be overlooked. Women's rights; ethnic minority rights; lesbian, gay, bisexual, and transgender rights; disability rights; patients' rights; children's rights; animal rights – these are all about protections and entitlements, about marking out a space of concern for this or that portion of society whose needs might otherwise be, and have been, overlooked. Political institutions can determine and protect these rights, but the demand for rights can emerge in the face of a tendency for the *polis* otherwise to overlook them. Fundamental human rights – to life, to privacy, to liberty, etc. – must also be safeguarded by a flourishing political community, whereas a malevolent political community might try to place them in jeopardy.

Living within diverse and complex communities of persons with values – valuers – who will wish to flourish in their different ways requires a political system to determine how the varied values of the political community are to be navigated and represented. Rights – and the duties that accompany rights (for both rights holders and duty bearers) – emerge in this political landscape. The political system must accommodate the rights of its citizens. But as we said at the start of this section, politics is about action. This can range from national policies about dementia to small-scale activities in local communities that can improve awareness of dementia, of the lives of individuals with dementia, and of their carers. So we are impelled from our metaphysical and ethical reflections to a political imperative to act. What is to be done? Well, it's with the values and rights of persons with dementia that we are concerned. But before we get there, we should take stock.

Persons, Values, Rights, and *Polis*

We have seen that metaphysics throws up a multilayered notion of situated embodied persons acting as agents in the context of interconnected narratives. Ethics draws on these underpinning notions but stresses the ways in which we, as human agents, can flourish as we strive to enact the things that have meaning and value for us. But we do this in the context of a complex political world of competing values, in which rights emerge as a way to protect our values and entitlements to basic levels of concern and regard within our political communities. This is the background to our public declaration, our Dementia Manifesto, and our call to action.

It is based, then, on these four main planks:

- **Personhood** – and the need for the broad view of our standing as situated embodied agents, interconnected and interdependent, who have narrative lives only understandable from just the biopsychosocial, spiritual, and uncircumscribable (i.e. uncontainable) perspective that is required for persons.
- **Values** – and the full view according to which facts are never simply facts but are always accompanied by evaluative judgements, so that values are ubiquitous and will be both shared and diverse, justified by underpinning conceptions of what constitutes the good life, which will, nonetheless, always be defeasible (always open to challenge) and to doubt and therefore require continual and careful scrutiny.
- **Rights** – and the correlative duties (where applicable) to ensure that the entitlements of all – even those with disabilities – are represented at the level of the *polis*, which must be a community of shared interests in human flourishing to achieve authentic human good where there is fairness, equity, equality, and justice within the institutions of the political community or state.
- *Polis* – we have used this term as our way of describing community and how we live our lives interconnectedly with others, not in isolation. This includes relationships involving dependencies, care, and support but also relationships involving expressions of ordinary human emotions, values, beliefs, and aspirations, as well as notions of citizenship, roles, and responsibilities. Rights are also a fundamental part of relationships in a *polis* but can affect people in different ways depending on a range of factors. Being aware of the ways in which rights can be part of how a *polis* functions requires knowledge and sometimes complicated balancing acts; but ignoring rights or dismissing them only creates greater dangers. And at times the *polis* may require, and can accommodate, challenges to the status quo and respond positively.

What Is to Be Done?

When Vladimir Lenin (1870–1924) wrote his political tract 'What Is to Be Done?', he borrowed the title from a novel written by an earlier Russian revolutionary, Nikolai Chernyshevsky (1828–1889). The need for some sort of revolution in connection with dementia care is very real given the demographic changes that are occurring worldwide. There are things that need to be done. Lenin's 'What Is to Be Done?' is credited to an extent with the creation of the Bolshevik party. For the sake of people living with dementia, we do now need to be 'Bolshie' though not quite in the way things occurred in revolutionary Russia! Our Manifesto is to do with how we live together in a world where people live with dementia and involves a social justice 'people's movement' that aims to accommodate a wide range of perspectives. In this context, we return to the three key principles which form our Manifesto and that we declared at the beginning of this chapter:

- *Dementia as humanity.* Dementia is a unique touchstone for understanding disease and disability, self-identity, aspects of the human condition such as ageing and mortality, a person's place in society, and how we live together as people, families, and communities. Appreciating both the expressed and implicit values of people living with dementia, those who provide support, care, and treatment for them, as well as how society values dementia, provides invaluable insights to who we are as people and how we relate to each other. At the same time, understanding and appreciating those same values, wherever possible, is essential to how we support people to live well with dementia, how we provide care and treatment for them, how we support those around them (both paid and unpaid carers), and how we educate the wider society about dementia. Dementia as humanity also reminds us that it is not a case of us (without dementia) and them (with dementia). Humanity is about us being 'all in it together': it's about solidarity. And we all have perceptions, experiences, and narratives about each other and conditions like dementia. VBP encourages us to be open and honest so that we become more aware of how an issue requiring action like dementia makes our own humanity a more explicit, collective, lived experience.
- *Dementia as disease and disability.* The first principle of our Manifesto, dementia as humanity, requires the coexistence of both themes – dementia as disease and dementia as disability – in theory and practice. People can conceive of dementia as a disease or a disability (or both), but not at the price of saying that one model should take priority over the other. This is also a requirement of VBP where one set of values should not be held up as 'right', excluding all others. Dementia is both a disease and a disability. This duality may at times be difficult to apply in situations that might involve decisions or dilemmas concerning individuals with dementia, right up to national policy making. But the duality is necessary as a principle in dementia care, and each model has benefits and can compensate where the other model is insufficient in a certain situation. Both have the potential to generate solutions and new ways of understanding dementia, now and in the future.
- *Dementia, VBP, and rights.* VBP provides an essential framework for providing support, care, and treatment to people with dementia and their families and friends. It is built upon an awareness and understanding of the values described in the first principle. Using VBP in partnership with evidence-based practice, along with an applied understanding of rights, will significantly enhance both the quality of life and the quality of care for people living with dementia.

These three principles that constitute our Manifesto run through the rest of this book like three threads, sometimes in parallel, sometimes interwoven. By reading the rest of this book, whoever you are, we hope it will lead you to take, individually or collectively, micro-actions in a mini-revolution. This should affect mainstream thinking, views, policy, practice, and lived experience regarding dementia.

References

Beauchamp, T. L. and Childress, J. F. (2001). *Principles of Biomedical Ethics* (5th edn). Oxford: Oxford University Press.

Hughes, J. C. (2011). *Thinking Through Dementia*. Oxford: Oxford University Press.

Hughes, J. C., Ingram, T. A., Jarvis, A., Denton, E., Lampshire, Z., Wernham, C. (2017). Consent for the diagnosis of preclinical dementia states: A review. *Maturitas*, 98: 30–34. http://dx.doi.org/10.1016/j.maturitas.2017.01.008

James, I. A. and Jackman, L. (eds). (2017). *Understanding Behaviour in Dementia that Challenges: A Guide to Assessment and Treatment* (2nd ed.). London and Philadelphia: Jessica Kingsley; pp. 280–92.

Jaworska A. (1999). Respecting the margins of agency: Alzheimer's patients and the capacity to value. *Philosophy and Public Affairs*, 28: 105–38.

Kitwood, T. (1997). *Dementia Reconsidered: The Person Comes First*. Buckingham, UK: Open University Press.

Nuffield Council on Bioethics (2009). *Dementia: Ethical Issues*. London: Nuffield Council. Available via: http://nuffieldbioethics.org/project/dementia/ (last accessed 2 January 2017).

Rights and Values Are Everywhere in Dementia!

Topics covered in this chapter
- This chapter is about rights and values and how prevalent they are in dementia care.
- Values are found everywhere in dementia care.
- These values come in many different forms, reflecting the different people involved.
- The stigma associated with dementia reflects the extent to which dementia is associated with negative values.
- Dementia is a condition which means that, by its nature, values are likely to be diverse and contradictory at times.
- Although there can be consensus, there is a real risk of diverse and conflicting values.
- VBP emphasizes the importance of taking deliberate steps to raise our awareness and increase knowledge of the values in play in any situation.
- Government and other initiatives, some from people with dementia themselves, mean that the stigma associated with dementia is gradually being eroded.

Take-away message for practice
You must always be aware that there are likely to be many values at play in any given situation. There is not necessarily one right decision, but it is more likely to be an acceptable solution if the values of all have been heard and understood.

Awareness and Knowledge

> 'Values are not always evident – like the air we breathe, we couldn't do without them, but because they are everywhere, they often go unnoticed.'
> *(Woodbridge and Fulford, 2004: 21)*

Introduction

In Chapter 2 we explained what we mean by values and why they are important. As we have seen, values-based practice (VBP) uses a very broad definition of the term 'values' that might loosely be described as 'action guiding words'. These include the things that are important for people (including people with dementia) in the way they make decisions and live their lives, for practitioners and staff to guide how they do their work, for how organizations operate, and for shaping wider society. They are also very important in relation to the law. In a democracy laws are perhaps the ultimate expression of the values that a society considers important.

As we shall see, this is important for several reasons in dementia care:

- Values can be found everywhere in dementia care and can be just as important in shaping decisions and action as scientific evidence – and sometimes they are more important or prevalent than scientific evidence.
- Using a broader definition of values can enable a shift away from the conflict that arises about whose values are 'right' and whose are 'wrong' when considering the best course of action in a given situation.
- Historically, however, certain values have dominated public and professional discourses on dementia in often quite negative and unhelpful ways.
- Values underpin rights, including legal rights, but in order to understand and apply these values correctly ('lawfully'), one must also have an awareness and basic understanding of the legal frameworks that are expressions of these values.
- Better-quality, more sensitive care can be provided by understanding the values that are 'in play' in any given situation, including where there are differences or conflicts involving values. For this to happen, however, everyone – especially practitioners – needs to be aware of these values.
- The first principle of our Manifesto, 'dementia as humanity', expresses our belief that dementia connects with values that include and yet go beyond a disease model approach to dementia care and involve fundamental issues concerning who we are as people and how we relate to each other. Values associated with understanding dementia as a disability may differ from those underpinning a disease model, but both can be used effectively in tandem.

Awareness and knowledge of values are therefore key to VBP. They are the starting point for a 'good process' in making decisions and taking action when providing care, support, and treatment in dementia care. This chapter explains how this awareness and knowledge can be achieved.

Values

Where Might One Find Values?

People express their values in the things they do, the decisions they make, and the way they lead their lives. This applies just as much to people with dementia as it does to anyone else, with or without a health condition. But we also express other values if we act in roles as practitioners, managers, carers, volunteers, citizens, etc. These values may be linked with a particular role but may also be the values of the organization we are working for and the community or society of which we are part. Organizations, in turn, may express values which reflect policies of national bodies such as governments. So values can be found from the personal level to the level of organizations and wider society. And they are also found in the law: as citizens, we express values by obeying the law (or express other values by not obeying it!).

Here are some sources of values and examples of where you might find them:

- *Personal values* – what's important to people in the way they make decisions and lead their lives, their beliefs and morals, how people expect to be treated and cared for, how people respond normally to being on the receiving end of rudeness, verbal abuse, or physical aggression. Apart from how people (e.g. service users, carers) express themselves in any given situation, other sources of personal values can be found in:

- · First-hand narratives and testimonies
- · Research reports
- · Media reports
- · Groups representing service users and carers

- *Practitioner values* – professional standards, codes of conduct
- *Practice values* – person-centred care, National Institute for Health and Care Excellence (NICE) guidelines
- Organizational values of service providers – mission statements, corporate values
- *Policy values* – outcome measures, personalization, 'dignity and respect' campaigns
- *Societal values* – laws, media stories

It is important to remember that people using health and social care services are neither professionals nor employees of those services and are likely only to express their personal values, although they will usually show respect for the law as well. People working in those services have to strike the correct balance between personal, professional, and organizational values, which at times is not easy because they may conflict. A very common source of tension, for example, is between values which emphasize personal autonomy or self-determination (ranging from expressions of personal preference through to principles contained in laws such as the Mental Capacity Act 2005 (MCA) and those that focus on duties of care, minimizing risk, and patient and public safety. An apparent tension may also exist between the values underpinning a disease model approach (focusing on treating and caring for the individual with dementia) and values associated with a disability model, which emphasizes how society should change to accommodate and support a person with dementia.

Of course, what people say they do or believe may differ from what they actually do or seem to believe in certain situations. As we have seen, and will recurrently see, people's expressed values (explicit values) may appear to conflict with the (implicit) values that guide their actual actions in particular situations (Colombo et al., 2003; Mental Health Foundation, 2009).

Awareness and Knowledge of Values Where There Is 'Values Consensus'

Some people might say that values are not important in healthcare because the real priority is to use science and medicine ('facts') to cure and treat people. If everyone agrees on the facts, then surely values don't really matter? Let's consider this with a vignette.

Vignette – Mr Abbott

Mr Abbott is 71 and lives in a large house with his wife. They own their home, and Mr Abbott deals with all the domestic finances. He enjoys watching sport and quiz shows on the TV, as well as gardening and driving. He used to play rugby and still enjoys going to his old rugby club to watch games and socialize. Over the last year he and his wife have noticed that he is finding it much harder to follow what's happening on the TV and find the right words when in conversation, and he has become confused or lost on several occasions when gardening or out driving. This is causing him a lot of worry, so with his wife he goes to see his general practitioner (GP). The GP refers him to the local memory clinic, run by Arcadia NHS Mental Health Trust. In the waiting room at the memory clinic there is a sign that says it 'aims to provide a swift, sensitive, and supportive service'. Over a period of a few weeks Mr Abbott has a number of tests and assessments, and all the staff are helpful and friendly. After three months Mr Abbott is seen by a psychiatrist at the clinic who tells him that he has Alzheimer's disease. The psychiatrist spends time discussing what this means with Mr and Mrs Abbott, the types of help and treatments available, and what Mr and Mrs Abbott can do to plan for the future. Although Mr Abbott is initially very upset, he finds the advice helpful and decides to 'make the most of it while he can', as well as to prepare for the future.

Mr Abbott is prescribed donepezil, which helps with some of the symptoms of the Alzheimer's. He is still able to drive and garden. He starts going to a local voluntary organization for people with dementia where he meets other people diagnosed with Alzheimer's and makes new friendships which are both supportive and enjoyable. He still goes to the rugby club and tells people he knows about his dementia diagnosis. They are sympathetic and supportive and encourage him to keep on coming, offering him help if he needs it. Mrs Abbott also gets advice and support from a family carers group. Mr Abbott decides to make a lasting power of attorney (LPA) for financial and property matters and makes his wife and eldest son, who lives nearby, his attorneys. Mr and Mrs Abbott contact local social services, but it is explained to them that they are not eligible for help because Mr Abbott's needs are not sufficiently severe and he would have to pay in any case, which Mr and Mrs Abbott understand and accept. However, Mr and Mrs Abbott are given a useful list of agencies providing home care, should they need them.

A year later, the Alzheimer's has gotten worse and staff from the memory clinic give Mr and Mrs Abbott more advice and support. Mr Abbott accepts that he has to stop driving and finds the gardening much more difficult. He makes an arrangement with his granddaughter, who has just learnt to drive, that she will come round once a fortnight and take him for a drive which he enjoys, and this enables her to practise her driving and also gives Mrs Abbott a break. Someone from the rugby club picks Mr Abbot up when there is a game on and drives him there and back so he can watch it. They employ a gardener, who agrees to do the gardening with Mr Abbott. He continues to meet with other people with dementia and they form a quiz group together. Mrs Abbott and the son register the LPA and they take over dealing with the domestic finances, although they continue to involve Mr Abbott as much as possible in this; any financial decisions affecting him which he lacks capacity to make himself they make in his best interests, in accordance with the MCA.

Commentary on Vignette
It may appear with the example of Mr Abbott that values are not particularly important. Mr Abbott is aware that he has a problem, seeks and obtains help for it, and a number of plans are put in place to enable him to live with the condition. This is similar to the experience of many people with physical illnesses and illustrates what Dickenson and Fulford (2001) describe as the 'fact and value' model of illness (see Chapter 2). On the surface, values do not appear to feature much in physical illnesses because there tends to be much greater consensus about the 'facts' of physical illness in terms of identifiable diseases, infections, and injuries and how these are experienced and described by people using similar ('objective') terms involving pain, symptoms, signs, and so forth. Likewise, there tends to be a consensus about the most appropriate treatment and interventions for physical illnesses (although these are constantly evolving as science and medicine develop).

Similarly, there are observable and agreed-upon 'facts' about Mr Abbott's Alzheimer's in terms of its symptoms, the problems these are causing him, the effectiveness of the care, and support and coping strategies that are put in place.

None of this, however, is to say there aren't values in play in this situation. Mr Abbott and his family are concerned about his health and want something done about it. The mission statement of the memory clinic is very 'value loaded' but seems to have been applied successfully in the case of Mr Abbott. The plans that are put in place enable Mr Abbott to continue to do the things that are important to him (that is, those things that he values), and the MCA is used in a way that is both lawful and helpful, again enabling him and the family to do things they judge to be of value. The response of people at the rugby club expresses human values. As a matter of common humanity, they express sympathy but also continue to acknowledge Mr Abbot as the same person he was before getting the dementia diagnosis, and they ensure that he can still be included and enjoy being part of the club. At a simple level they also respond to Mr Abbot's dementia as a disability; people adapt their behaviours to accommodate Mr Abbot, rather than expecting him to change. So in reality, a lot of values are being expressed, guiding decisions and actions, but crucially these are congruent across all the individuals and organizations involved. In other words, there is a consensus of values (which includes Mr Abbott's values) concerning what is happening and the best ways of dealing with the situation. This consensus therefore supports the 'facts' of Mr Abbott's Alzheimer's and the best ways to respond.

Awareness and Knowledge of Values Where There Is Values Diversity or Conflict ('Dissensus')

Where everyone (including, as far as possible, the person living with dementia) is in agreement about the right decisions or courses of action to be taken, then there are likely to be aligned or shared values, and there is no particular need to pay close attention to those values. However, the origins of VBP partly derive from situations involving people using mental health services where a consensus of values, or indeed facts, often does not exist. This can occur for several reasons:

- Mental health problems and conditions (including dementia) affect people's emotions, thoughts, moods, cognitive abilities, communication, beliefs, feelings, and so on. The subjective experience of a condition like Alzheimer's will therefore differ enormously from individual to individual. The way people express their values in responding to a problem or condition will both affect and be affected by it in ways unique to the individual. Imagine if Mr Abbott insisted on continuing to drive after it was clear it was no longer safe for him to do so.
- Some people may not experience a mental illness or condition as distressing or causing difficulties and therefore not see any need for help or support. Indeed, they may have other explanations for what is happening, actively reject or resist any offer of help or support, or seek it in different ways. A person may want people around them to accept and adapt to their condition, viewing it as a disability rather than a medical problem which needs 'fixing'. Values of self-determination, self-definition, and autonomy, and perhaps societal changes, are important to the individual, whereas care or treatment may be the priority for those around them. Imagine if Mr Abbott denied there was anything wrong with

him, refused to go to the GP or memory clinic, rejected any help or support, or started blaming TV broadcasters, other drivers, etc., for causing him problems.

- For the reasons noted earlier, the 'facts' of a mental health problem or condition can be significantly less clear than they are in physical diseases – subjective experience and human agency play a much greater part in the observable symptoms and behaviours, as well as in the possible responses and interventions.

- Some people using mental health services, and health and social care more widely, have found them unhelpful, discriminatory, or oppressive. The values of the service or people working for them have not been congruent with the values of the service user or family carer, or they simply don't provide the help that is being sought. Imagine if the memory clinic or GP had told Mr Abbott his diagnosis, said there was no effective treatment, and just told him to come back when things got worse; or imagine if other organizations Mr and Mrs Abbott approached were reluctant to help because he had dementia.

- A condition like Alzheimer's can make people very vulnerable, especially if their legal rights are not understood or are not respected. Imagine if Mr Abbott's son thought that being an attorney meant he could spend Mr Abbott's money as he wished, or if Mr Abbott's granddaughter started using Mr Abbott's car without asking him.

- Conditions such as dementia have historically been poorly understood in society, generated fear, and acquired stigma. People with a dementia diagnosis have often experienced being shunned or excluded by friends and even family members simply by virtue of having the diagnosis, irrespective of how it actually affects them. Imagine if Mr Abbot's granddaughter was fearful of getting in the car with him or the rugby club no longer made him feel welcome.

It is easy to see how situations like these involve people choosing different courses of action based upon what they believe to be 'right' or 'wrong' (or both). Underlying these actions are values. Conflict can arise about whose values are 'right' and whose are 'wrong'. Sometimes these conflicts may be expressed explicitly by people arguing using terms such as 'autonomy' versus 'duty of care'; sometimes the argument may be framed in terms such as 'wanting to be at home and not in hospital' versus 'protecting the patient'; or expressed as 'I don't want people to treat me differently and I want to be included' versus 'he had better stop doing that because he isn't safe or might cause embarrassment'. But all of these phrases or words express values.

Where there are these kinds of differences, VBP emphasizes the importance of taking deliberate steps to raise our awareness and increase knowledge of the values in play, in order to improve understanding and ensure that responses, decisions, and actions are better informed and take into account, as far as possible, all the values in play. The importance of understanding, respecting, and upholding people's rights and the different legal frameworks that may apply add another dimension which requires compliance but also provides help and protection in many situations.

Another vignette can help to illustrate this.

Vignette – Mrs Barber

Mrs Barber is a 77-year-old widow and lives alone in a flat. She has a daughter who lives locally and visits regularly and a son who also lives nearby with a large family but whom she does not see very often. A year ago Mrs Barber was diagnosed with early-stage Alzheimer's disease. There have been several mishaps at home, with kettles boiling dry and muddles over food (which has gone off) and appointments. She has also had a series of falls. Two weeks ago Mrs Barber had a further fall while out shopping and fractured her hip. She was admitted to a general hospital where she had surgery which was successful. Her rehabilitation programme has gone well, and she has recovered her mobility although she needs to walk with a cane. Although at times she has been confused, believing the hospital to be a hotel, she has had capacity to give consent to her treatment and rehabilitation and is now expressing a wish to go home. The hospital she is in is run by the Shangri-La NHS Trust, whose mission statement is 'each patient is unique and safely treated with care, dignity and respect'.

The staff treating Mrs Barber also want her discharged as soon as possible because of a lack of beds but think that she should go into a care home rather than return to her own home. Mrs Barber is entitled to help from the local authority, and they agree with the hospital that she should go into a care home. The local authority's social services mission statement is 'promoting wellbeing, independence, safety, and individualized care and support'. They have identified a care home nearby that has a room available and is willing to take her. The care home is run by the Xanadu Care Group, whose mission statement is 'high-quality care provided in a safe, respectful and dignified manner'. Mrs Barber's son agrees with the hospital and social services because he wants her 'kept safe'.

However, Mrs Barber has made it clear that she wants to return to her own home. Her daughter supports Mrs Barber in her wish to return home and says that, even if social services won't help Mrs Barber, she will ensure that Mrs Barber has the support she needs to manage at home. Although the hospital wants Mrs Barber discharged as soon as possible, they say they are not prepared to discharge her back home – the hospital considers it a safeguarding issue and have said that it is in Mrs Barber's best interests that she should go to the care home because she has dementia. An independent mental capacity advocate (IMCA) has become involved and is questioning whether the hospital is using the Mental Capacity Act correctly.

Commentary on Vignette

Imagine if you worked for the local community mental health team and were responsible for coordinating Mrs Barber's care. The vignette illustrates the importance of being aware and knowledgeable about all the values in play, including how they are expressed through use of the law, which would include:

- Mrs Barber's values in terms of the importance of returning to her own home, supported by her daughter, and ensuring that others involved in her care adapt the situation to her wishes. If one considers the situation in terms of 'person-centred care' (albeit another values-laden concept), Mrs Barber's values should be the ones that have primacy and everyone should be working in ways to fulfil them. Even if Mrs Barber lacked capacity, values expressed by service users in research studies together with policy guidance emphasize the importance of helping people return to their own home wherever possible. In the UK there is also legal precedent for this (see the case of Manuela Sykes in Box 4.1). Although hospital discharge is an everyday routine for staff, it is a very significant event for Mrs Barber, particularly given that it could represent a major life change if she were to go into the care home – this difference in the values attached to discharge must also be recognized.
- The values being expressed by the hospital and social services focus on safety, risk, safeguarding, and perhaps a concern about being blamed if something goes wrong. Although stated fairly explicitly in relation to Mrs Barber, these are also somewhat implicit values, as they are not very consistent with the mission statements of the organizations (though all the organizations have safety as an explicit value). Some staff are likely to have genuine concerns about Mrs Barber returning to her own home – these will be expressed as professional concerns, but it may also be that they have personal concerns, perhaps because they themselves have a relative with dementia (it is also often true that those hospital staff who have not worked in the community are

not aware of what is possible in terms of viable support). For many general hospitals, possible neglect of patients is a source of great concern following the report into the Mid-Staffordshire hospitals in the UK where patient neglect led to excessive numbers of patients dying (HM Government, 2013). On the other hand, corporate values focusing on speedy discharges is a tension pulling in the other direction.

- Values associated with safeguarding appear to be driving the use of the MCA – it is not clear if Mrs Barber lacks capacity to make the decision to go home. A diagnosis of dementia is not sufficient proof of a lack of capacity. If she does not lack capacity, then a best interests decision cannot be made on her behalf even if her wish to return home is considered to be an unwise decision (Emmett et al., 2013). However, the hospital seems to be trying to use best interests as a way of addressing their safeguarding concerns. Although the Care Act of 2014 places adult safeguarding on a statutory basis, decision making around mental capacity is still governed by the MCA. This creates potential tension between values expressed in two different laws. It is crucial to be aware of the rights and values expressed in both pieces of legislation in order to decide on a course of action. As Williamson and Daw point out, VBP can help when ensuring practice is in keeping with laws like the MCA (Williamson and Daw, 2013, especially pp. 107–8).
- It is possible that the explicit values expressed by Mrs Barber's son are not the same as his implicit values. It is possible that he wants to use his mother's flat for a member of his own family. Although most families are wholly supportive of the person and desire his or her best interests, abuse is most commonly committed by people who know the person who is being abused, and people with dementia are particularly vulnerable.
- It is also worth considering an alternative scenario where Mrs Barber has an LPA which authorized her daughter to make decisions about her health and welfare if Mrs Barber lacked capacity to make them herself. If Mrs Barber lacked capacity to agree to being discharged, her daughter could act on her behalf by refusing to consent to a move into long-term care and support her to return home on the basis that it was in Mrs Barber's best interests. However, this could escalate the situation and result in the hospital making a safeguarding referral.
- Awareness and knowledge of values should not be treated as an abstract philosophical or ethical exercise, nor are they wholly dependent upon professional knowledge about dementia or the law. Mrs Barber's wish to return to her own home needs to be considered in the context of her dementia. But medical and legal factors can distract from her human desire to express her identity and be in familiar surroundings. Together with her daughter's support, the views of her son and those of the staff involved in the scenario indicate the relevance of our principle of 'dementia as humanity', combining biopsychosocial factors (and values) with expressions of identity, place, and relationships.

This vignette illustrates the importance of being aware and knowledgeable about the values that are in play in situations like these, both explicit and implicit, as well as a person's rights. In some respects, the issues associated with applying these aspects of VBP in dementia care are similar to issues in other areas of health and social care. However, as we will see in the next section, particular factors need to be considered in relation to dementia, particularly historical and condition-specific issues, to supplement awareness and knowledge of values, and rights, that are applied in situations like these.

Box 4.1 The Case of Manuela Sykes

Westminster City Council v. Sykes [2014] EWCOP B9 (24 February 2014).

Manuela Sykes (1925–2017) was a political campaigner all of her life. She was diagnosed with dementia in 2006, and she made a living will. For her, the main thing was the quality of her life, not the length of it. In 2011, she made a lasting power of attorney, in which she stated: 'I would not like my attorney to sell my property. My wish is to remain in my own property for as long as this is feasible'.

It was difficult for local services to support her. She refused care at times. There were confrontations, but also evidence of self-neglect and worries about hygiene and the safety of her property. Manuela had lost weight, had been found wandering, and seemed unaware of issues to do with her personal safety. In October 2012 she was detained in hospital under Section 2 of the Mental Health Act (MHA).

Acting in what was considered to be her best interests, the authorities discharged her to a nursing home, where her deprivation of liberty was authorized. But Manuela persistently opposed living in the care home and stated her wish to move back to her own home, where she had lived for 60 years. The local authority asked the Court of Protection to review matters.

District Judge Eldergill fully understood why the authorities were nervous on behalf of Ms Sykes about her going home. Nevertheless, he was also clear that she was deprived of her liberty: 'Patently she is not free to go home or visit her home, and the state claims legal power to control her liberty and movements indefinitely, and not simply to define a place of residence for her; therefore she has been deprived of that usual liberty which the rest of us enjoy. No aspect of her liberty of movement remains under her own control'.

The Court went to see Manuela Sykes in the nursing home and considered the issue of her 'best interests' very carefully. The judge noted: 'It is her welfare in the context of *her wishes, feelings, beliefs and values* that is important. This is the principle of beneficence which asserts an obligation to help others further their important and legitimate interests. In this important sense, the judge no less than the local authority is her servant, not her master' (emphasis added).

The judge recognized that there would be problems with her going home, but he weighed matters up thus:

> Several last months of freedom in one's own home at the end of one's life is worth having for many people with serious progressive illnesses, even if it comes at a cost of some distress. If a trial is not attempted now the reality is that she will never again have the opportunity to live in her own home. Her home will be sold and she will live out what remains of her life in an institution. She does not want that, it makes her sufficiently unhappy that sometimes she talks about ending things herself, and it involves depriving her of her liberty.

Accordingly, the judgment allowed that Manuela should return home on a trial basis.

Another important point in this hearing was that Ms Sykes was named, whereas normally, where a person lacks capacity, the Court would protect his or her anonymity. But Manuela Sykes said that she wanted to be named and the judge felt that this was in keeping with her long-held political views, that she would want transparency to allow proper understanding and publicity around the issues that were being considered. These were, after all, issues that touched on basic human rights to do with liberty and autonomous decision making in matters to do with one's private life, and these were the sort of issues that Manuela Sykes had felt passionately about all of her life.

Values and Dementia

The word 'dementia' is derived from the Latin *de* (without) and *mens* (mind). It's an umbrella term to describe a set of symptoms associated with a number of specific illnesses, including Alzheimer's disease, the most common form of dementia. Other common types of dementia include vascular dementia, dementia with Lewy bodies, and fronto-temporal degeneration (see Hughes 2011). As such, it has often been seen as (at best) a confusing term and (at worst) unhelpful and pejorative, especially to those diagnosed with dementia. Until relatively recently, describing people with dementia as 'demented', 'mentally infirm', or even as 'vegetables' was quite common, even though similarly pejorative terms had largely disappeared for other groups with cognitive impairments, such as people with learning disabilities.

Dementia was also a condition that until the end of the twentieth century rarely featured in public policy debates about health and social care. In 1999, the Department of Health published a 153-page National Service Framework (NSF) for Mental Health – a strategy and plan (with financial resources attached) to improve mental health services for adults up to the age of 65 in England (Department of Health, 1999). It did not include dementia. In 2001, the Department of Health published a 202-page NSF for Older People (defined as being aged 65 and over), which included a chapter on mental health (Department of Health, 2001). Contained within this chapter were five pages on dementia. This NSF came with no additional financial resources.

Historically, therefore, the lives of people with dementia and the services that supported them were considered of little value in public policy terms. Low rates of diagnosis (partly for reasons of 'therapeutic nihilism' – 'what's the point of diagnosing if no treatment can be offered and the prognosis is so grim?') and the tendency only to diagnose late in the condition meant that people with dementia were either ignored or were too cognitively impaired to have a voice, let alone express what was important to them. Images of frail old people sat nodding or dribbling in care homes was the defining stereotype of people with dementia. They were seen to be virtually 'value-less'. Although dementia was heavily defined in medical terms and there was little controversy about diagnosis, as compared to the more contested terrain of 'functional' mental illnesses, it was seen as a disease of hopelessness with no possibility of cure, recovery, or treatment. This process of dehumanizing the person with dementia and their experience of living with the condition, often observed in the way others (including professionals) treated them, was (as mentioned in Chapter 1) described by the highly influential researcher and writer Tom Kitwood as 'malignant social psychology' (Kitwood, 1997).

Over the last 10–15 years in the UK this picture has changed dramatically. The exponential increase in the numbers of people with dementia; the growing voice of family carers, professionals, and organizations representing them; and the work of people like Kitwood, together with a series of high-profile reports about the poor state of services for people with dementia (for example, National Audit Office, 2007), led to the publication in 2009 of a national dementia strategy for England (with financial resources attached), and the other UK countries quickly followed suit (Department of Health, 2009). Although there is still no prospect in sight of a cure or effective treatment for the major forms of dementia, such as Alzheimer's, virtually every organization delivering health or social care has dementia on its radar. For example, at least 25 per cent of all hospital beds in the UK are occupied by patients over the age of 65 with dementia, even though most are admitted to hospital for other reasons, such as falls (Alzheimer's Society, 2013). In 2012, the prime minister published a dementia 'challenge', which included the creation of 'dementia-friendly communities' to enable people with dementia living in them to be better supported (Department of Health, 2012).

Policy has therefore evolved rapidly, and inevitably this has meant that the sources and range of values that can be observed in dementia care have expanded dramatically. At the same time laws such as the Adults with Incapacity Act of 2000 (Scotland), the MCA (which covers England and Wales), and the Care Act (which covers England only) have come into force. These laws, and similar laws in other jurisdictions, have created a further nexus of legal rights, entitlements, and values directly relevant to people with dementia.

Yet for several reasons, it is not as simple as just seeing dementia as if it were playing catch-up with other cognitive and mental health conditions, as we shall see.

Hearing the Voice and Values of People with Dementia

Finding out what people with dementia are experiencing and what is important to them should be at the centre of any interaction by practitioners, but this has frequently not been the case, partly for the reasons indicated earlier. Low rates of diagnosis (especially early diagnosis), the progressive effect on cognition and communication, and many family carers asserting that they could speak on behalf of their relative with dementia (and collectively on behalf of people with dementia) meant that the person's voice, or a wider 'service user' narrative, was still struggling to be heard (indeed, the term 'service user' is not much used in dementia). This was in stark contrast to the fields of learning disabilities and mental health problems, where there has been a long-standing and effective service user voice challenging particularly what has been viewed as an overly medical model.

Awareness and knowledge of the values of the person with dementia, whether as individuals or collectively, was extremely limited. Quality-of-life studies of people with dementia, for example, usually depended upon proxy reports by family carers or professionals, but there is increasing evidence that family carers in particular tend to project their own quality of life onto the life of the person with dementia, which does not always accurately reflect the experience of the person with the condition (Alzheimer's Society, 2010).

Recently this has begun to change, with a growing number of individuals publishing their own stories of living with dementia (see, for example, Davis, 1989; Jennings, 2014; Whitman, 2016), with research carried out to collect the views of people with dementia (Pratt and Wilkinson, 2001; Williamson, 2008), and with the rise of dementia 'activist' groups led by or actively involving people with the condition, such as groups that are part of the UK Dementia Engagement and Empowerment Project network (DEEP) (Williamson, 2012). These initiatives provide invaluable sources of information about what is important to people with dementia and feature increasingly in policy documents (see, for example, the statements describing the expectations of people with dementia and carers in the National Dementia Action Alliances Dementia Declaration[1]).

Although there remains a significant challenge in finding ways of getting information from people in the later stages of the illness, approaches using different communication techniques, such as 'Talking Mats', have achieved some success (Murphy and Oliver, 2013). Legally recognized instruments, such as written statements and LPAs, also provide a means for people in the earlier stages of dementia to record their wishes, beliefs, values, and preferences whilst cognition and communication are still fairly intact.

However, unlike the more radical groups of people with mental health problems, who challenge the very concept of mental illness and diagnosis, or many people with

---

[1] www.dementiaaction.org.uk/nationaldementiadeclaration

learning disabilities who advocate for a human rights–based approach using the social model of disability (requiring change in society's attitudes and responses to people with disabilities, rather than locating problems of disability in the individual), most dementia activists to date have neither challenged the concept of dementia nor campaigned for a more rights-based approach. A notable exception to this is Scotland, where the Scottish Dementia Working Group (made up of people with dementia) have worked with the Scottish government to produce a Charter of Rights for People with Dementia and Their Carers (Alzheimer's Scotland, 2009) and a human rights–based approach to developing Scotland's dementia policy.

Dementia: Still a Disease of Despair?

Despite the increased attention given to dementia, societal values still frequently have an excessively negative skew and pejorative tone. Consider these recent media headlines:

- 'Alzheimer's: A living death' – *The Daily Mail Online* 27 March 2012
- 'Britain unprepared for 'tsunami' of dementia patients' – *The Independent* 16 September 2012
- 'Dementia is a modern-day plague which robs people of their identity and dignity' – *The Daily Mirror* 11 December 2013
- 'Listen to those who care for dementia sufferers' – *The Daily Telegraph* 14 October 2014

The values contained within these headlines may well invoke fear or pity but offer nothing positive to people with dementia. Most of the terms, including the word 'sufferers', are ones towards which people with dementia have expressed their dislike (Dementia Engagement and Empowerment Project, 2014) and contrast dramatically with the 2009 dementia strategy, which had the title of *Living Well with Dementia*.

Dementia: Medically Diagnosed But Lacking a Medical Response

Despite the greatly increased focus on dementia, including additional resources for research into its different forms (especially Alzheimer's), there is still no cure or universally effective treatment for any form of dementia. Although there is a growing number of nonpharmacological interventions for dementia, the evidence base for these is still limited. Again, this is in contrast to functional mental health problems where there is a significantly greater evidence base for a range of different treatments, including drugs and psychological interventions (though drug treatments are disliked by many service users, particularly because of side effects). In other words, there is much less 'values consensus' about what works best for any particular individual as an effective intervention for dementia (especially regarding nonpharmacological interventions) despite the objective (organic) nature of various types of the condition, as shown by brain scans (which paradoxically cannot be used clinically to diagnose psychoses such as schizophrenia). Where consensus around effective evidence-based interventions for dementia is less clear, values become central. In addition, the growing influence of rights-based approaches to dementia has resulted in an increased focus on understanding dementia as a disability and the importance of interventions aiming to change how individuals and society at large adapt in order to accommodate people with dementia (Mental Health Foundation, 2015). However, this also means that a diversity of values is almost intrinsic to how people cope with their dementia or care for people with dementia.

Box 4.2 Person-Centred Care

This guideline offers best-practice advice on the care of people with dementia and on support for their carers. There is broad consensus that the principles of *person-centred care* underpin good practice in the field of dementia care and they are reflected in many of the recommendations made in the guideline. The principles assert:

1. the *human value* of people with dementia, *regardless* of age or cognitive impairment, and those who care for them
2. the *individuality* of people with dementia, with their *unique personality* and *life experiences* among the influences on *their response* to the dementia
3. the importance of the *perspective* of the person with dementia
4. the importance of *relationships and interactions* with others to the person with dementia, and their potential for promoting well-being.

The fourth principle emphasises the imperative in dementia care to consider the needs of carers, whether family and friends or paid care-workers, and to consider ways of supporting and enhancing their input to the person with dementia. This is increasingly described as *'relationship-centred care'*.

© NICE (2006; updated 2016) CG42: *Dementia: supporting people with dementia and their carers in health and social care.* Available from www.nice.org.uk/guidance/cg42 All rights reserved. Subject to Notice of rights.

NICE guidance is prepared for the National Health Service in England. All NICE guidance is subject to regular review and may be updated or withdrawn. NICE accepts no responsibility for the use of its content in this product/publication.

The centrality of values in dementia care is reflected in clinical guidelines for practitioners working in the field. NICE, the body that determines what treatments and interventions are cost-effective for different illnesses and conditions, published its clinical guidelines for dementia in 2006 (NICE, 2016). This opens with the text in Box 4.2 (in which we've added italics) and includes Kitwood in its references. It also highlights the relevance of the MCA, the importance of involving carers, non-discrimination in service provision for people with dementia, and the importance of coordinating health and social care. None of these should be seen as controversial, but what they do illustrate, as the italics show, is how important values are in dementia care. Of particular note are the second and third principles, which emphasize that understanding a person's personality, perspective, and biography is key in influencing the way dementia affects them and how they respond to it; in other words, the importance of subjective experience and human agency in the 'facts and values' model of Dickenson and Fulford (2001).

However, the more limited evidence base in dementia care, caused partly because of the limited effectiveness of pharmacological and other health interventions and the diversity of values, also creates difficulties in terms of being sure one is aware and knowledgeable of all the possible values in play in a given situation. It also throws the field wide open to a plethora of other possible interventions and responses. There are currently far too many to list, but here is a sample of some better-known ones:

- Assistive technology
- Doll therapy
- Life story work
- Multisensory environments

- Namaste care – an end-of-life care programme
- Outdoor adventure activities
- Paro – a therapeutic robot baby harp seal
- Participatory arts and drama
- Peer support groups
- Pet therapy
- 'Reading for the brain'
- Reminiscence therapy
- 'Singing for the brain'
- Specialised Early Care for Alzheimer's (SPECAL)
- Sudoku and crossword puzzles
- Swimming

Evidence for the efficacy of these interventions varies but tends to be quite limited, although those involved in delivering the interventions are usually keen to promote the benefits. Clearly some will coincide with values held by the person with dementia (or their carer) and are therefore likely to contribute to the person's sense of wellbeing, if nothing else. Yet the challenge of being aware and knowledgeable about the interventions themselves and the values that underpin them is clearly enormous.

Dementia: Shifting Values

The third reason why being aware and knowledgeable of values in dementia is different from other fields is the effect that most forms of dementia have on a person's personality. Dementia is neither an episodic nor stable condition. Although some of its cognitive aspects are similar to some learning disabilities, all forms of dementia involve progressive changes and deterioration in a person's functions. Most commonly this involves memory loss, extreme confusion, problems in communicating, or believing one is living in a different reality (which may be caused by cognitive difficulties, such as disorientation, or by actual 'delusions'). In addition, there are changes in behaviour, such as becoming very disinhibited or responding to hallucinations, which also occur quite frequently in some forms of dementia. The underlying changes, which reflect brain pathology, cannot be reversed, and although many people with dementia will have periods of lucidity and be orientated in time and place, these do not last and usually become less frequent as the condition progresses.

As we shall see elsewhere in this book, these changes pose a variety of challenges, an obvious one being that it becomes harder for the person to communicate what is important to them, what they are feeling, or what they need. In addition to any recorded statements by the person themselves, close family and friends are likely to be the best source for awareness and knowledge of the person's values, including more intuitive knowledge of what may defuse or trigger distress or agitation for the person. This 'tacit' (or 'craft') knowledge may also be very important in understanding expressions of physical pain or discomfort when the person is unable to communicate this through words or gestures (Hughes, 2014).

Perhaps more challenging is being aware and having knowledge of a person's values when the dementia seems to result in fundamental changes to a person's personality, self-identity, sense of time and place, behaviour, and perception of others – and the values that go with these changes. This can be illustrated with a vignette.

Vignette – Mr Czacki

Mr Czacki is 82 and has been diagnosed with vascular dementia. Two years ago, he moved into a care home because his wife was unable to continue looking after him in their own home. Mrs Czacki tries to visit Mr Czacki every day, although the severity of his vascular dementia means that he finds it increasingly hard to remember who she is. There is no indication that he has ever been unfaithful to his wife. Three months ago, Mrs Davis moved into the care home. Mrs Davis is 83, a widower, and has Alzheimer's. Shortly after moving into the home Mrs Davis struck up a friendship with Mr Czacki. This developed into a more intimate relationship involving holding hands and cuddling each other. Mrs Davis describes Mr Czacki as her boyfriend. Mrs Czacki became very upset the first time she visited Mr Czacki and found him with Mrs Davis. Mrs Czacki asked the staff to try and stop them from being together. The staff said they would do their best and would certainly ensure that Mr Czacki and Mrs Davis are not together when Mrs Czacki visits, providing Mrs Czacki rings the home half an hour before she plans to visit. Mrs Czacki agrees to this and is able to see Mr Czacki without Mrs Davis being around. However, Mrs Czacki notices a change in Mr Czacki's mood – he seems more distracted and grumpy, keeps on asking who Mrs Czacki is, and asking for 'that other woman'. Meanwhile staff are very concerned about Mrs Davis because every time they separate her from Mr Czacki before Mrs Czacki visits, Mrs Davis gets extremely upset and agitated and physically tries to resist being separated. Even after she has been separated from Mr Czacki she continues to be distressed, shouting and crying, and is physically hostile towards staff. Some staff think that she should be prescribed medication to keep her calm, but other staff are very resistant to this and think they shouldn't be separating Mr Czacki and Mrs Davis. Most staff agree that the current arrangement is not working.

Commentary on Vignette

Situations like this pose major challenges to being aware and knowledgeable of the values in play.

- Are the values that Mr Czacki's behaviour is indicating just symptoms of his dementia or are they now his 'real' values? Even though it seems reasonable to link the change in his behaviour to the effect of the dementia, this still doesn't mean that the 'values' that underpin the behaviour can be changed. It should also be acknowledged that people's personalities, with or without dementia, can in any case continue to change over time, and this can lead to changes in lifestyle, relationships, and so forth. Furthermore, as with many health conditions, the subjective experience of having the illness, beyond the symptoms themselves, can cause changes in a person's personality. Likewise for Mrs Davis, how far do her current values relating to relationships reflect her premorbid values?

- Are Mr Czacki's and Mrs Davis's behaviours expressions of unmet needs in terms of intimacy, affection, and companionship that nearly all humans seek and which, because of his situation, cannot now be met for Mr Czacki, at least not easily by Mrs Czacki? Living in unfamiliar surroundings, perhaps aware of becoming more confused but not necessarily understanding why, might all be additional reasons for seeking comfort and support from another.

- Mrs Czacki's values and emotions are very important to take into consideration. She clearly finds the situation upsetting, and she is likely to feel that she is losing her husband not just to an illness but also to another woman. However, Mrs Czacki is not disabled by cognitive impairment and therefore is more able to understand and possibly even be supported to adapt to the situation.

- In the absence of any clear evidence base for knowing what to do in these situations, the response will be dictated by values based upon professional experience and knowledge, as well as the everyday practice of the care home. However, it may be hard for some staff to separate their personal values about, for instance, fidelity in relationships from their professional values in deciding what to do.
- If the agreed response by the care home staff was not to challenge or try to reorientate residents to reality in these kinds of situations, this would mean that certain values came into play, which might include:
  - Respecting residents' wishes and preferences;
  - Collusion with, adapting to, or 'going along with' certain situations to minimize distress;
  - An emphasis on 'dementia-orientated reality' over truth telling and reinforcing actual reality;
  - Providing intensive support and information to Mrs Czacki to try and help her come to terms with the effect the dementia has had on Mr Czacki;
  Or perhaps it might indicate just a very laissez-faire, nonconfrontational, 'path of least resistance' type of care.
- If the response had the reverse focus (i.e. staff would normally try and prevent these situations arising through distraction, separation, and close supervision, or by trying to reorientate the person), then other values would appear to be in play, which might include:
  - Respect for the wishes and feelings of the family;
  - A determination to maintain more traditional moral integrity in the approach to care (i.e. the importance of honesty and fidelity);
  - A belief that Mr Czacki's behaviour could be changed and that Mrs Davis's interest in Mr Czacki (and the distress caused by separating them) would subside over time.
- In both situations, a knowledge of dementia, but also perhaps of people's rights, would be needed:
  - The importance of promoting wellbeing (a concept which appears in the UN Declaration of Human Rights as well as some national legislation) and the loss of factual but not emotional memory associated with dementia (i.e. Mr Czacki cannot remember who Mrs Czacki is but can retain a sense of comfort derived from close relationships) mean that it will be detrimental to both Mr Czacki's and Mrs Davis's wellbeing, at least for a period of time, to try and keep them apart.
  - Do Mr Czacki and Mrs Davis have capacity to make the decisions that are leading them to want to be with each other? If they do, then their decisions have to be respected. If they do not, then what is in their best interests (remembering to take into account Mrs Czacki's views in this as well)? How could it be ensured that best-interests decisions were agreed upon and carried out consistently?

Conclusions and Key Points

- Values are extremely prevalent, but also very diverse in dementia care, partly because the contributions from science and medicine to knowledge of how to deal with most forms of dementia are much more limited compared with many other health conditions.
- Until fairly recently, there has been very limited information from people with dementia about what is important to them, individually and collectively, but this

is changing. This can be seen as representing a move from the disease model of dementia towards a disability model, where the rights of the individuals concerned are given prominence in keeping with the slogan: 'Nothing about us without us!'
- Most forms of dementia pose very significant challenges in relation to how a person's values may change quite dramatically during the course of the illness.
- Awareness and knowledge of relevant legal frameworks – in their own right expressions of values – are essential in any given situation, and these frameworks can be very helpful in clarifying aspects of VBP.

References

Alzheimer's Scotland (2009). *Charter of Rights for People with Dementia and Their Carers in Scotland.* Available via: www.alzscot.org/assets/0000/2678/Charter_of_Rights.pdf (last accessed 19 December 2017).

Alzheimer's Society (2010). *My Name Is Not Dementia. Literature Review.* London: Alzheimer's Society.

(2013). *Counting the Cost. Caring for People with Dementia on Hospital Wards.* London: Alzheimer's Society.

Colombo, A., Bendelow, G., Fulford, B., and Williams, S. (2003). Evaluating the influence of implicit models of mental disorder on processes of shared decision making within community-based multi-disciplinary teams. *Social Science & Medicine* 56, 1557–70.

Davis, R. (1989). *My Journey into Alzheimer's Disease: Helpful Insights for Family and Friends.* Wheaton, IL: Tyndale House.

Dementia Engagement and Empowerment Project (2014). *Dementia Words Matter: Guidelines on Language about Dementia.* Available via: http://dementiavoices.org.uk/wp-content/uploads/2015/03/DEEP-Guide-Language.pdf (last accessed 19 December 2017).

Department of Health (1999). *National Service Framework (NSF) for Mental Health.* London: Department of Health.

(2001). *National Service Framework (NSF) for Older People.* London: Department of Health.

(2009). *Living Well with Dementia: A National Dementia Strategy.* London: Department of Health. Available via:

www.gov.uk/government/publications/living-well-with-dementia-a-national-dementia-strategy (last accessed 19 December 2017).

(2012). *Prime Minister's Challenge on Dementia: Delivering Major Improvements in Dementia Care and Research by 2015.* London: Department of Health. Available via: www.gov.uk/government/publications/prime-ministers-challenge-on-dementia (last accessed 9th October 2018)

(2016). *Prime Minister's Challenge on Dementia 2020; Implementation Plan.* London: Department of Health. Available via: www.gov.uk/government/publications/challenge-on-dementia-2020-implementation-plan (last accessed 19 December 2017).

Dickenson, D. L. and Fulford, K. W. M. (2001). *In Two Minds. A Casebook of Psychiatric Ethics.* Oxford, UK: Oxford University Press.

Emmett, C., Poole, M., Bond, J., and Hughes, J. C. (2013). Homeward bound or bound for a home? Assessing the capacity of dementia patients to make decisions about hospital discharge: Comparing practice with legal standards. *International Journal of Law and Psychiatry* 36, 73–82.

HM Government (2013). *Report of the Mid Staffordshire Foundation Trust Public Inquiry. HC 947.* London: The Stationery Office. Available via: www.gov.uk/government/publications/report-of-the-mid-staffordshire-nhs-foundation-trust-public-inquiry (last accessed 19 December 2017).

Hughes, J. C. (2011). *Alzheimer's and Other Dementias: The Facts.* Oxford, UK: Oxford University Press.

(2014). *How We Think About Dementia: Personhood, Rights, Ethics, the Arts and What They Mean for Care.* London and Philadelphia: Jessica Kingsley Publishers; pp. 151–64.

Jennings, L. (ed.) (2014). *Welcome to Our World.* Canterbury, UK: Forget-Me-Nots.

Kitwood, T. (1997). *Dementia Reconsidered.* Buckingham, UK: Open University.

Mental Health Foundation (2009). *Model Values? Race, Values and Models in Mental Health.* London: Mental Health Foundation. Available via: www.mentalhealth.org.uk/sites/default/files/model_values.pdf (last accessed 19 December 2017).

(2015). *Dementia, Rights and the Social Model of Disability. Policy discussion paper.* London: Mental Health Foundation.

Murphy, J. and Oliver, T. M. (2013). The use of Talking Mats to support people with dementia and their carers to make decisions together. *Health and Social Care in the Community* **21**, 171–80.

National Audit Office. (2007). *Improving Services and Support for People with Dementia.* London: The Stationery Office. Available via: www.nao.org.uk/report/improving-services-and-support-for-people-with-dementia/ (last accessed 19 December 2017).

NICE. (2016). *Dementia: Supporting People with Dementia and Their Carers in Health and Social Care. [Clinical Guidelines 42].* London: National Institute for Health & Care Excellence. Available via: www.nice.org.uk/Guidance/CG42 (last accessed 19 December 2017).

Pratt, R. & Wilkinson, H. (2001). *Tell Me the Truth* London: Mental Health Foundation. Available via: www.mentalhealth.org.uk/publications/tell-me-truth (last accessed 19 December 2017).

Whitman, L. (2016). *People with Dementia Speak Out.* London: Jessica Kingsley Publishers.

Williamson, T. (2008). *Dementia – Out of the Shadows.* London: Alzheimer's Society.

(2012). *A Stronger Collective Voice for People with Dementia.* York, UK: Joseph Rowntree Foundation.

Williamson, T. and Daw, R. (2013). *Law, Values and Practice in Mental Health Nursing. A Handbook.* Maidenhead, UK: Open University Press.

Woodbridge, K. and Fulford, Bill (K. W. M.). (2004). *Whose Values? A Workbook for Values-Based Practice in Mental Health Care.* London: The Sainsbury Centre for Mental Health.

Legal case

Westminster City Council v. Sykes [2014] EWCOP B9 (24 February 2014).

Reasoning about Values

Topics covered in this chapter

- Conceptual thought is required to decide between right and wrong, good and bad, in particular contexts.
- We need to expand the horizons within which we determine what is right or wrong, good or bad.
- The big three ethical theories are consequentialism (utilitarianism), deontology, and virtue ethics.
- There are also various other approaches to ethical difficulties: principlism, casuistry, care ethics (feminist ethics), communicative ethics, hermeneutic ethics, and narrative ethics.
- The framework from the Nuffield Council on Bioethics is useful in discussing real cases and does itself reflect values.
- Values awaken ethical concerns and encourage a broader view.
- In discussing ethics, therefore, we inevitably touch upon principles that underpin clinical practice.
- But we are also able to highlight the three principles of our Manifesto:
  - *Dementia as humanity*
  - *Dementia as disease and disability*
  - *VBP for dementia plus rights.*

Take-away message for practice

Our sense and awareness of values is a sense and awareness of ethics. We must look at cases one by one and in some depth, keeping in mind fundamental principles such as solidarity and the importance of personhood. A broad view of the person will help to encourage the correct understanding required by ethics.

Introduction

The process of VBP brings values to the fore. In the last chapter, we saw that values are everywhere and that they may be diverse. We have therefore already raised a question about how conflicting values are to be settled. If, for instance, one person values autonomy highly and so thinks that the autonomous wishes of an individual should be honoured, whereas someone else thinks that the values of behaving in accordance with the norms of society are more important, how are we to decide between these competing values without seeming to be arbitrary?

To make this more concrete, think of a person with mild-to-moderate dementia who wishes to continue to drive, who highly values the independence that comes from driving, as opposed to the professional who feels that greater weight should be given to the protection of the public, that is, who values public safety higher than the individual's autonomy. Now in response to this, someone might say that the apparent conflict can be sorted out in a practical, factual manner. The person with dementia can simply go to a driving assessment centre and his or her driving can be assessed against objective standards. Indeed, this is probably the way in which such a matter would be handled. It does not, however, get rid of the conflict in values.

The person with dementia might be failed at the driving assessment centre if he or she, when tested on the open road, joins a dual carriageway too slowly. But it is important to see that values are at play here. If I join a dual carriageway at 20 miles an hour when the average speed on the road is 70 miles an hour, it is undoubtedly true that I am unsafe and could be called a social nuisance. Why, however, should we accept that the average speed on the dual carriageway should be 70 miles an hour? And what if my speed was 40 miles an hour? At 40 miles an hour, it might still seem that I am a nuisance to the person who is already on the dual carriageway and travelling at 60, let alone 70, miles per hour. Yet travelling at 40 miles an hour onto a dual carriageway does not seem to be outlandish. And what about 35 miles per hour? And so on! No one would wish to deny that certain driving practices are simply too dangerous to be acceptable. But what is or is not acceptable is itself determined by social values, which can vary considerably among individuals and different social groups. Nowadays, for instance, people are actually taught to drive faster, whereas this has not always been the case. The individual's autonomous wish to continue driving, where autonomy is valued, comes up against a different set of values. Why should one person's values trump another's? This question leads us to the content of the present chapter, which is to do with reasoning about values.

However, there are significant strategic difficulties when reasoning about values, because we might all have slightly different opinions about how to proceed. To some extent, these opinions will reflect our different intellectual commitments. It could, for instance, reasonably be argued that if we wished to look at how to reason about values, we should undertake a sociological study. In other words, we might wish to go out onto the streets to conduct surveys or to organize focus groups to determine what values people actually hold and the extent to which values are shared or diverse. Or perhaps someone would say that we should look at the law, which (after all) codifies our values but which itself might involve different value commitments that wait to be adjudged by the courts. Our approach in this chapter is to use the tools of philosophical ethics. In other words, we acknowledge that the conflicts in terms of values will, in practice, have to be decided by actions that may be deemed to be right or wrong, good or bad. But our further commitment is to the thought that right or wrong, good or bad, must be decided on the basis of conceptual thought. So this is philosophical ethics.

Our second major commitment is to the idea that we shall do well here if we expand the horizons within which we determine the best course of action to take. The horizons within which values are seen and negotiated must be broad if we are to do the right thing for people with dementia and their carers. This is because values are themselves pervasive, and talk of people's values forces us to consider the nooks and crannies of people's lives in all of their complexity.

Ethical Theories and Approaches

In deciding whether something is right or wrong, good or bad, philosophers have tended to rely on three major ethical theories:

- **Consequentialism:** The rightness or wrongness of an action depends on its consequences. According to the proponents of utilitarianism, which is the best-known of the consequentialist theories, an action is right insofar as it maximizes happiness or pleasure and wrong insofar as it causes unhappiness or pain. Equally, we could argue that the consequences of an action have to maximize welfare, or anything else which we thought was of sufficient value to determine which actions were good – the point simply being that we have to look at the consequences of our actions before we judge them morally.

- **Deontology:** These moral theories suggest that some actions should be done largely irrespective of their consequences and others must not be done despite any desired consequences, because certain actions *just are duties* (the term comes from the Greek *deon*, which means a duty). According to deontologists, some actions will seem right or wrong in themselves. So deontological theories are often seen as contradicting consequentialism, because the deontologist will sometimes say that, whatever the consequences, some things (such as, perhaps, telling lies) should never be done.

- **Virtue ethics:** A good action is the one which a virtuous person would do, and a virtuous person is the one who, because they have the virtues (or natural dispositions), will flourish or do well as a human being. That is, you do well as a human being if you are honest, compassionate, just, brave, and so forth. Virtue ethics encourages us to think about what it is to be a good human being before we start looking at our duties or the consequences of our actions.

Of course, there is much more to be said about each of these theories. Hundreds of books have been written about them. Almost inevitably, some theorists argue that these three large schools of thought are not actually as distinct from each other as their proponents would have us believe. Each of these theories can, however, be useful in thinking about particular problems in connection with dementia. Take, for instance, the dilemma to which we have already alluded, that of whether or not to tell someone the truth (see the case of Mrs Emery overleaf). In connection with dementia, this has recently become a hot topic (James et al., 2006; Culley et al., 2013; Williamson and Kirtley, 2016).

Other Approaches

One such approach, well known in the field of medical ethics, is to use the four principles. This is sometimes known as **principlism**. The four principles are as follows:

- Beneficence – doing what is good
- Non-maleficence – avoiding what is harmful
- Autonomy – allowing self-rule
- Justice – distributing goods or resources fairly

The four principles of biomedical ethics were developed by Beauchamp and Childress (2008) as a way to capture some of the insights of the three major ethical theories in a

Vignette – Mrs Emery

Mrs Emery is a 78-year-old lady who has a mixed vascular and Alzheimer's type of dementia. She has been living at home with her husband who is physically ill. He has joked in the past that she provides the brains and he provides the brawn. Mrs Emery knows that she has to look after her husband and he can remind her what to do for them both. In this way they have managed for several years. But Mr Emery falls ill and is admitted to hospital. The family are not able to cope with their mother, so she goes into a care home for respite. She accepts this, having been told that it is a little holiday for her because she has been working so hard. She seems relatively settled in the care home. Occasionally she becomes anxious about her husband, but she is reminded that she is only there for a short while and that she will be back to look after her husband once the holiday is over. Sadly, however, Mr Emery dies whilst in hospital. The family try to break this news to their mother, but when they even suggest that he is very unwell, she becomes extremely agitated and determined to leave the care home. So they back down, do not go on to say that he has died, and instead say that he is picking up and that she should continue to enjoy her short break. The staff in the care home are asked to employ the same tactic and not to say that Mr Emery has died but just to say that he will be out of hospital soon and that she should enjoy her rest. The hope is that gradually she will forget to ask, because she does seem to be settling very well in the care home as long as she is given suitable reassurance. However, there are some staff in the care home who do not feel it is right to tell Mrs Emery lies, whereas others agree with the family that the key thing is her wellbeing, which they think is better served by what may seem a small 'white lie'.

Commentary

Each of the three main ethical theories can provide a useful commentary on the case of Mrs Emery. We should notice straightaway the extent to which the theories prescribe or proscribe particular courses of action:

- **Consequentialist** arguments would often be used in such a case as this to support the view that it is better to tell Mrs Emery a small lie than to tell her the truth. Of course, one objection to this is that the lie in question, namely that her husband is alive rather than dead, is rather a large lie! But the consequentialists can argue that if you do one thing, namely tell her the lie, she remains reasonably content and happy, whereas, if you tell her the truth, she becomes extremely agitated and upset. In which case, they would say, it is obvious that you should tell the lie. But there are further things for the consequentialists to think about. For a start, no one has actually yet told Mrs Emery the truth, that her husband has died, because the family only got as far as telling her that he was very ill. Of course, she might wish to leave the care home if she believes her husband is very ill, because she has been his carer. But if she were told the full truth, namely that he had died, perhaps after a period of understandable grief, she would again settle and would realize why she did not need to leave the care home. In other words, it is possible that the truth might have good consequences. Against this, another consequentialist might yet say that she would have to be retold the news of his death every time she questioned why she was in the care home and, if she forgot meanwhile, each of these new revelations would be extremely upsetting for her so, again, the good consequences of lying might be supported. Alternatively, however, there is another type of consequentialist who would be inclined to ask what the consequences will be if, having told a lie to Mrs Emery, it starts to seem easy to tell people with dementia all sorts of lies, or even to start to tell lies to other people. If telling lies were to become *the rule*, or the norm, it might be that the consequences for society would eventually be so bad as to outweigh the possibility that lying could be a good thing. Thus, consequentialists, or utilitarians, might argue this way or that, but they would have an inclination to tell a small lie if the consequences were obviously going to be good.

- On the whole, the **deontologist**, is going to be steadfastly against lying. Deontologists would say that we have a duty to tell the truth, plain and simple. They could give a more sophisticated account of this by arguing that it would be irrational to say that something was good if its general adoption could not be sanctioned. To this extent, the deontologist is a little like the utilitarian who looks at the consequences of something being adopted as a rule. However, the deontologist is not looking primarily at the consequences, but at the nature of our obligations as rational human beings. It would not be rational, they would argue, to do something to someone else which we would not wish to have done to us – not because of the consequences, but just because this does not make sense. It certainly does not seem to be just. So the deontologist would tend to be against lying to Mrs Emery. Nevertheless, there are problems for the deontologist, because it can also be said that we have a duty to care for the person. It might be argued that you cannot properly care for Mrs Emery if you are persistently upsetting her and making her agitated by forcing the truth upon her. Deontologists, therefore, might also argue amongst themselves about exactly what to do in the case of Mrs Emery, but they could feasibly reach a position which suggested that the duty to care for her could be realized by distraction rather than by truth-telling. They could argue that distracting her or changing the subject would avoid the lying but would allow them to continue to care for her. Nevertheless, some deontologists might still object to this and insist that it would simply be playing with words to think that a deceit (or avoiding telling the truth by saying something to distract the person) was not a lie, and they might persist in saying that we can only really care for her if we are being completely honest with her.

- The **virtue ethicist** will neither think about particular duties nor rely solely on the consequences of actions, but will instead analyse the situation in terms of the virtues. Again, there are some ways in which the conversation of the virtue ethicists might mirror that of the deontologists. There is obviously the virtue of honesty, but (as for the deontologist) this is likely to conflict with the virtue of compassion. Unlike the deontologist, however, the virtue ethicist can draw on a broad array of virtues to push forward the discussion. For instance, there is the virtue of bravery. One of the possible psychological reasons for avoiding telling Mrs Emery the truth is that it will be uncomfortable and even frightening to see her reaction. In this way, virtue ethics looks inward to the dispositions that allow someone to act in certain ways and not in others. There is also the virtue of fidelity – being true to the person – which will not be possible if we are being dishonest. It could be argued, too, that one relevant professional virtue is that of being steadfast, which entails consistency and dependability, which may be undermined by a lack of truthfulness. Perhaps the most useful virtue is that of practical wisdom, which is sometimes called prudence. This involves knowing how to achieve the end at which you are aiming. Practical wisdom is something which is acquired over years through education and practice. It allows the practitioner to see how to take things forward. The difficult thing for the virtue ethicist is to give an account of how all of these varying virtues can be put into effect at once. Is it possible to show charity whilst being honest? Would not distraction, even if this is a form of deceit, be more charitable than complete honesty? There is an interesting point to note about virtue ethics. The other two theories, if fully embraced, might leave you feeling that you had done a good thing. If you have maximized happiness by telling the lie, or done your duty by telling the truth, you might then feel that you could give yourself a pat on the back on the grounds that, according to your preferred theory, what you had done was good, right, and proper. But the experience of the virtue ethicist would be wholly different. Perhaps I feel that the virtuous person must in this case tell the truth, but if I am virtuous then my compassion will still leave me feeling distraught on behalf of Mrs Emery. Or, alternatively, prudence might dictate some form of deceit, yet as a virtuous person I will be left with the feeling that I have not shown great charity, perhaps, and have not acted with fidelity.

We see, therefore, that the three main ethical theories give us a lot to think about and provide tools for the analysis of ethical dilemmas, which includes giving us a vocabulary to discuss the ethical aspects of situations we might encounter, but also do not provide us with unequivocal answers. Each of the theories can be used to give a clear-cut answer, but any such answer can be challenged using the same theory, and can then be challenged further by one of the other theories. It is partly for this reason that other ethical approaches have sometimes seemed more appealing than the well-established grand theories of ethics.

Table 5.1 Examples of ethical approaches to dilemmas in practice

Ethical approach	Description
Care ethics	This is a development of feminist ethics, which stresses the importance of relationships, where care itself and the nature of care are important in deciding what is right or wrong.
Communicative ethics	This approach suggests that if we get the communication right, then the right decision will follow.
Hermeneutic ethics	According to this approach, what is required is the correct interpretation in a given context, where the meaning of actions is understood properly so that the right response is forthcoming.
Narrative ethics	The rightness or wrongness of an action will become apparent in the context of the details of the story, but this will entail understanding the stories of all those involved.

manner that would be readily usable by clinicians on the shop floor. But as Table 5.1 shows, there are various other approaches to ethical issues.

Only a few examples of the ethical approaches are given in Table 5.1, but much more can be found out about these approaches elsewhere (Hughes and Baldwin, 2006; Hughes, 2013). Suffice it to say that when the various ethical approaches are added to the ethical theories, we are presented with a rich conceptual toolbox with which to consider ethical difficulties in connection with dementia. The value of the ethical approaches, which have by and large been developed more recently, is that they stress the importance of individuals in a context, where the context itself is relevant to the decisions that may or may not have to be made. These ethical approaches, therefore, not only increase the vocabulary with which we can discuss cases, they also expand the horizons in the sense that they give us not just different perspectives on the same view but also new views to consider at the same time. Thus, not only might we think about the relevant virtues and the consequences of an action, but we will now also think about the relationships between the main actors in the narrative that is being played out.

All of this leaves us with two further questions which we wish to pursue in this chapter. First, how do we actually decide between the competing ethical theories and approaches?

It is all very well having an expanded view, but when faced by a dilemma, how do we decide which way to go? Second, so far we have left unsaid anything about the direct connection between ethics and values. It is all very well seeing values as pervasive, in the same way that we can think of ethics as infiltrating every aspect of our human interactions or practice in connection with people with dementia, but what is the relationship between ethics and values?

Processes and Frameworks for Clinical Decision Making

As we have seen in Chapter 1, values-based practice itself presents a process that helps to navigate difficult decisions when there are clashes of values. In doing this, it also outlines a process that will be useful in dealing with ethical dilemmas. It might have been thought that ethical dilemmas could be solved by the application of ethical theories. But as we have seen, there is relatively little chance that an ethical theory as such will provide a clear-cut and incontrovertible solution. The nuance added by the sort of approaches we have described, which involve attention to context and relationships (amongst other things), suggests that the process of solving ethical dilemmas will require more engagement with the concrete circumstances of particular cases. An example of a practical clinical ethics framework for approaching clinical ethics dilemmas can be found on the website of the United Kingdom Clinical Ethics Network (UKCEN) (www.ukcen.net/index.php/education_resources/support_guide/section_c_ethical_frameworks). (This is discussed more fully in Hughes [2013]: pp. 732–735.) There is, however, a framework for approaching ethical issues which is more specific to dementia that can be found in the report of the Nuffield Council on Bioethics (2009) entitled *Dementia: Ethical Issues*. The ethical framework in this report highlighted six components, as shown in Table 5.2.

Both the UKCEN framework and the Nuffield Council's framework adopt a **casuist approach** to ethical analysis. That is, they emphasize the importance of thinking about the details of the individual case. This allows us to see that each case will inevitably be different. Many cases will be broadly similar, of course, but in one case the person with dementia might also have other serious physical difficulties (e.g., heart and kidney failure); whilst in the next case there may be a very large family, all of whom are actively involved in the care of the person with dementia; and then again, in a further case, the person with dementia may have written out in great detail, with the help of a solicitor, what his or her wishes would be under particular circumstances. The differences between similar cases may be quite small but nevertheless big enough to alter the potential decisions that have to be made. In each case the relevant values will differ. Case-based reasoning, therefore, emphasizes the facts. It also starts to point towards a process. First of all, the facts need to be established very clearly. But second, these facts in themselves start to suggest what might be morally relevant, and this, in turn, might direct us towards the approach that we should take. There is still the requirement that our moral or ethical approach should be justifiable, which includes making sure that any terms used in the arguments put forward are clearly defined and are used coherently, as well as that the argument itself should be valid: that is, the conclusions of the argument follow from the premises and the premises themselves are true or justifiable.

But as we have already seen in Chapter 2, where there are facts, there are invariably values! It is noticeable that the Nuffield Council's framework (Table 5.2), in describing its case-based approach to ethical decisions in Component 1, talks about identifying the

Table 5.2 An Ethical Framework for Dementia

Component 1	A 'case-based' approach to ethical decisions: Ethical decisions can be approached in a three-stage process: identifying the relevant facts, interpreting and applying appropriate ethical values to those facts, and comparing the situation with other similar situations to find ethically relevant similarities or differences.
Component 2	A belief about the nature of dementia: Dementia arises as a result of a brain disorder and is harmful to the individual.
Component 3	A belief about quality of life with dementia: With good care and support, people with dementia should be able to expect to have a good quality of life throughout the course of their illness.
Component 4	The importance of promoting the interests both of the person with dementia and of those who care for them: People with dementia have interests, both in their autonomy and their well-being. Promoting autonomy involves enabling and fostering relationships that are important to the person and supporting them in maintaining their sense of self and expressing their values. Autonomy is not simply to be equated with the ability to make rational decisions. A person's well-being includes both their moment-to-moment experiences of contentment or pleasure and more objective factors, such as their level of cognitive functioning. The separate and different interests or concerns of carers must be recognized and promoted.
Component 5	The requirement to act in accordance with solidarity: The need to recognize the citizenship of people with dementia and to acknowledge our mutual interdependence and responsibility to support people with dementia, both within families and in society as a whole.
Component 6	Recognizing personhood, identity, and value: The person with dementia remains the same equally valued person throughout the course of their illness, regardless of the extent of the changes in their cognitive and other functions.

(From: Nuffield Council on Bioethics [2009] Box 2.1, p. 21.)

relevant facts but immediately moves on to speak about the interpretation and application of appropriate ethical values to those facts. And Component 4 speaks of supporting people 'in maintaining their sense of self and expressing their values'. This is not, however, the end of values in this framework. Component 6, for instance, is about recognizing the personhood of the individual, which helps to maintain identity and value. That is, the idea of being a person is immediately tied to the idea of value.

Indeed, underpinning the expanded horizons within which we must view ethical dilemmas, which we established earlier in this chapter, is a broader view of what it is to be a person with dementia. We discussed this broader view in Chapter 3 (see also Hughes, 2001; Hughes, 2011), but it can be summarized by saying that the person should be thought of as a situated embodied agent. The key notion here is that of being situated. This places the person within an individual context, but one which cannot be entirely circumscribed. For it involves the whole person's history, biological and psychological make-up, social and cultural background, ethical and religious or spiritual beliefs, geographical and juridical boundaries, friendships and relationships, hobbies, and political interests. Some of these are empirical matters, and some are evaluative (and they also influence each other). In some cases, the person with dementia may also have 'time-shifted' so the facts and values that are important to them may not be ones that relate to the present time (such as the person appearing to believe they are a younger version of themselves living in a different era).

Some years ago, there was an important debate around whether 'critical interests' or 'experiential interests' were more salient for the person with dementia. Dworkin (1993) argued that critical interests should be given more weight. These are the sort of important interests that shape the life of a person as a whole. Dresser (1995), on the other hand, stressed the importance of experiential interests, which were those things that were important to the person immediately in the context of their present experiences. This debate was sometimes phrased in terms of a conflict between the 'then-self' and the 'now-self'. But for our purposes we wish to note that the crucial thing is that this debate was about values. What are the values that have shaped a person's life against what might be of value to him or her right now? In commenting on this debate, Jaworska (1999) pointed out that the key thing was to recognize that the person with dementia is a *valuer*. In other words, the person has and continues to value things. This is a move that in itself helps to broaden the horizon, because the values of the person, then and now, are seen within a single perspective. To put it another way, our values are embedded within our lives. Some may remain very important, some become less so. Then and now are not two separate, dichotomous places, and in demonstrating this, dementia teaches us something about our humanity generally. *Dementia as humanity* is key to our Manifesto: we learn about ourselves in thinking about dementia, about the saliency of those values that are extended across our lives but which can also change. There is thus something organic about our values and how they should be evaluated. Taking a broad view of the person, therefore, sets before us a great variety of facts and values, which will need to be weighed up very carefully.

To return to the question about how we actually decide between competing ethical theories and approaches, it starts to look as if it need not be that decisions are either consequentialist or deontological, and it need not be that someone must prefer narrative ethics rather than feminist ethics. The casuist approach allows quite openly the possibility that we can choose the ethical theory or approach which best suits the dilemma we are facing. The sort of framework commended by the Nuffield Council on Bioethics in Table 5.2 similarly encourages us to keep in mind not just the casuist approach but various other beliefs about dementia and some underpinning concerns – for instance, the need for solidarity. And we should continue to recognize the important role that personhood must play in our thoughts. But central to all of this is that we should promote the interests both of the person with dementia and those who care for the person (Component 4), which itself entails an openness to the values of all concerned. So the answer to the question 'how do we decide?' is that we decide by taking the broadest possible view. Our decisions are made no less rational by such an approach, as long as we pay attention to the need for clear and coherent arguments and rational thought. But the approach will bring in a broader array of concerns, including facts but also emotions, inclinations, stories, *and values*. VBP also encourages a broad view, and it allows input from the various moral theories and approaches we have been discussing, in keeping with the third of our Manifesto principles.

Applying the Frameworks

Before answering our second question, which was about the relationship between ethics and values, we shall now return briefly to reconsider the cases set out in Chapters 2 and 4 in the light of our thoughts concerning reasoning about values.

Vignette – Mr Abbott

Mr Abbott, you may recall, was the man who gradually developed memory problems and was given the diagnosis of Alzheimer's disease. Some of his day-to-day skills were eroded, including his ability to drive, so he had to give this up. There were, however, no major dilemmas in all of this because, as we saw in Chapter 4, the values were largely shared.

If we look again at Table 5.2, especially at Component 4, we can see that the case of Mr Abbott demonstrates very well the ways in which both the autonomy and the wellbeing of a person can be promoted. Mr Abbott was able to continue to pursue his hobbies and interests, whilst at the same time he was supported in ways which were enabling. His wellbeing was promoted, but the interests of those around him were also taken into account by the way, for instance, that his granddaughter was able to drive him places, which was good for him, good for her, and good in terms of public safety. The use of a lasting power of attorney in the case of someone such as Mr Abbott enables him to maintain a sense of agency and thereby a sense of citizenship. In this way, he continues to express his values and is enabled to do so by a sense of solidarity (Component 5 in Table 5.2). Throughout all of this, Mr Abbott's personhood is recognized and he continues to be equally valued, regardless of the extent of the changes that are occurring because of his dementia. This is the second principle from our Manifesto: *dementia as disability and disease*. Mr Abbott's citizenship, supported by the solidarity of those near to him and by society itself, does not ignore the fact that he has a disease, but fosters a sense of his rights. As a disabled person, he still shares the same rights enjoyed by the rest of the *polis*.

In a slightly different scenario, it would be easy to imagine that some of the issues might not be dealt with in quite such an open manner. The immediate effect would be to bring into conflict the values of the various people involved. Perhaps, for instance, attempts could be made, behind the back of Mr Abbott, to make sure that he no longer drives. This need not be done in a malicious way. It might be thought that it would save him from embarrassment. As we saw towards the start of this chapter, it would be possible to put forward consequentialist views to support either being honest with him about the driving or dishonest. But it would be easy to imagine a consequentialist argument that would lead us into problems with Mr Abbott. Much better, therefore, to take the broad view, which brings into focus more sharply the values of Mr Abbott and of his family.

Vignette – Mrs Barber

Mrs Barber is the lady with Alzheimer's disease who has been admitted to hospital following a fall and a fracture of her hip. But once in hospital, a question is raised about her ability to cope at home and, in part because of pressure on beds, it is suggested that it would be in her best interests for her to go into a care home. She and her daughter are opposing this. There seems to be a supposition that she lacks the capacity to make this decision and, therefore, it is reasonable for the hospital to act in her best interests. We have already seen in Chapter 4 that this case displays a variety of conflicting values.

There is, in theory, a straightforward legal solution to the dilemma, which is to seek a definitive statement concerning whether or not Mrs Barber has the required capacity. If she does have the capacity to make a decision about whether or not she goes home or into a care home, then her decision (according to the MCA which applies in England and Wales) should hold sway. The difficulty, however, is that decisions about where we should live are heavily value-laden (Greener et al., 2012). So even identifying the relevant facts can be difficult. We must then apply ethical values to those facts (Component 1 of Table 5.2), which is also difficult. Some of the facts will form the basis of the information which Mrs Barber will be required to understand, recall, and weigh up if it is to be said that she has the capacity to make the relevant decision. But the question of which bits of information she should be able to recall itself involves value judgements. Judgements will also have to be made about the sort of quality of life that Mrs Barber can expect back at home and in a care home. But this places an onus on social services to ensure that the right sort of support is available so that Mrs Barber can enjoy a good quality of life, despite her dementia (Component 3 of Table 5.2).

Again, the scenario could be changed slightly. If, for instance, the stress for her daughter were going to be huge if Mrs Barber went home, then this would have to feature in our estimation of the interests both of Mrs Barber and her daughter. In this case, however, Mrs Barber's autonomous wishes and her daughter's wishes coincide so that her interest in well-being (Component 4 of Table 5.2) will be promoted as long as the right support is in place. The question of solidarity (Component 5 in Table 5.2) can be understood in terms of citizenship. As a citizen, Mrs Barber deserves and should receive appropriate support to allow her to live her life in the way that she wishes to, as long as this is not causing too much upset for others and thereby curtailing their own interests and ability to act as useful citizens. Furthermore, the idea of citizenship can be used to question whether care at home or institutional care is better as a means to enabling the sort of participation that goes along with citizenship. And, to repeat, this way of thinking emphasizes the rights of those with disabilities rather than their disease status: *dementia as disease and disability*. Finally, in Component 6 of the Nuffield Council's Framework (Table 5.2), we need to understand Mrs Barber in a rounded manner as a person whose identity in some part depends on *place*, where this is not just a geographical but also a psychosocial concept. The importance of home, therefore, is stressed. Understanding the importance of home for Mrs Barber is also to understand her values and to support her personhood: *dementia as humanity*.

The case of Mrs Barber seems to hinge upon legal interpretation (of whether or not she has capacity, for instance), but it also epitomizes the tension between risk and safety. The implementation of the MCA in England and Wales was criticized by the House of Lords in 2014 because it was said that social service departments were too risk averse and clinicians were too paternalistic. There is undoubtedly some truth in these accusations. But it is important to note that in being both risk averse and paternalistic, professionals are simply reflecting certain sorts of values which appear to dominate social thinking. It may well be that the value placed on safety and avoiding risk is too great when it comes to people such as Mrs Barber. But it should also be recognized that part of the difficulty is that *value judgements are required throughout the process of assessing someone's capacity*. What is then important is that all of the values in play should be given the right amount of consideration: *VBP for dementia plus rights* (the third principle of our Manifesto). A broad view is more likely to make this occur. The broad view brings into focus the diverse and conflicting values so that the need to mount a case or develop an argument for the precedence of one person's values over those of another is plain to see. Moreover, the broad view allows a greater range of theories, approaches, moral arguments, and evaluative judgements to be considered in a manner which chimes with the richness of our moral lives.

Vignette - Mr Czacki

Mr Czacki is the 82-year-old man with vascular dementia from Chapter 4 who has formed a relationship with Mrs Davis, who has Alzheimer's disease, in the care home where they now live. This is greatly upsetting for Mrs Czacki when she comes to visit her husband. But it is also upsetting for Mrs Davis when she cannot be with Mr Czacki.

One of the tactics used in casuistry (see Component 1 in Table 5.2) is to compare the current situation with other similar situations in order to look at ethically relevant similarities or differences. So, in this case, we could ask what the situation would be if neither Mr Czacki nor Mrs Davis had a living spouse. Ethical concerns might still be raised if, for instance, it was felt that one of the two did not have the capacity to consent to any form of sexual intimacy. We should note, therefore, that there is a legal perspective. In the present case, however, this does not seem to be to the fore. Even if neither partner had a living spouse, we could imagine that there might yet be concern expressed by offspring. Let's explore the hypothetical situation that Mrs Czacki is no longer alive. It may be that some of the children would then wholly approve of the relationship, given that their parents seem to be happy. But it is easy to imagine that some children might be very upset or disgusted by the relationship. This helps to show us that there is an emotional perspective to be considered. However, there may be more to this than simply emotions. It may be that some of the children would think that Mr Czacki's critical interests were not served by his present relationship if, for instance, in the past he has avoided relationships with women since the (hypothetical) death of his wife. It may be that he thinks Mrs Davis is his wife and his children feel that if he were aware of his mistake, he would be disgusted with himself. It may be that his devotion to the memory of his wife, which reflects his faithfulness to her, has shaped the latter stages of his life so that his children feel his present relationship is in some sense inauthentic. But other children might take a more experiential view and feel that what he values now is of more importance than what he might have valued in the past. As we have said earlier, the broad view of the person, which incorporates the person's values throughout the individual's life, should enable some sort of weighing up of what is of importance in the current situation. Perhaps previous faithfulness to his wife has, after all, blocked Mr Czacki from enjoying other things that he has always valued. Perhaps, for instance, he stopped socializing in certain sorts of ways or dropped hobbies which he had previously enjoyed.

Alternatively, it is at least conceivable that Mr Czacki, on the basis of deeply held religious views, might determine to live out his life in a celibate manner following his long and fulfilling marriage. Perhaps there are circumstances under which these values seem to be so important in the life of a man who has been guided by deeply held religious convictions, that they would outweigh what appear more ephemeral experiential interests. In other words, what is required is careful and considerate thought about the values of those involved, which is encouraged by thinking of the relevant similarities and differences in different scenarios. The distress of Mrs Davis when she is parted from Mr Czacki might be overridden by the level of contentment that Mr and Mrs Czacki derive from each other's company when Mrs Davis is not in the picture. But if Mr Czacki is also extremely distressed and this is not alleviated by the presence of Mrs Czacki, then it is harder for staff to ignore. The values of the staff must also come into the equation. In saying this, we are also alluding to several of the other components set out in the Nuffield Council's Framework (Table 5.2). We would be trying to promote Mr Czacki's autonomy but recognizing that he stands in relationship to Mrs Czacki. In addition, however, we would be trying to promote his wellbeing, which is increased by 'moment-to-moment experiences of contentment or pleasure' (Component 4 of Table 5.2). Meanwhile solidarity requires that we should try to support all involved, which points towards an open process of discussion, with the values of everyone being considered in the ways that values-based practice would suggest (as set out in Chapter 1). And, finally, all of this is underpinned to some extent by recognizing the personhood of those involved, which is why we must take all of their values throughout their lives into consideration insofar as this is possible.

In Hughes, Beatty, and Shippen (2014) a number of different scenarios to do with sexuality in dementia were discussed and the elements of values-based practice were applied. The conclusion of that discussion was as follows:

> Ethical issues around sexuality in the context of dementia are difficult because of the conflicting values that emerge. Our own attitudes towards sexuality and to sexual relations are often at issue and, given that these are frequently intensely private, confronting conflicting values in an overt manner presents problems. Nevertheless, it seems important that sex and sexuality should be regarded and dealt with at the level of underpinning values given the centrality of these issues to our lives.... A values-based practice approach is a way to bring into the open the values that support or inhibit intimacy. Sexual intimacy may be unwanted or inappropriate for a variety of reasons, but it should not be regarded as routinely problematic when it otherwise provides the possibility of authentic human flourishing.
>
> (Hughes, Beatty, and Shippen 2014: pp. 236–237)

Ethics and Values

We also wished to say something about the connection between ethics and values. What is the relationship between these two?

One thing we have seen in the previous section is that clinical scenarios, especially where there is conflict, but even when there is not, always involve values as well as facts. We have also seen that values can guide clinical practice. It is by paying close attention to the values of all concerned that we are more likely to reach an outcome that is as acceptable as possible. There are two further points to be made.

First, values *as such* are neither right nor wrong. We may value one sort of music more highly than another, but the fact that Jack likes jazz and Jill likes Renaissance music is a matter of preference, not of ethics. We might say, therefore, that values are wider than ethics in that they extend to needs and wishes. So far, then, we have agreed with the conclusions of Chapter 1 of *Essential Values-Based Practice* (Fulford, Peile, and Carroll, 2012, p. 9):

- Values are wider than ethics.
- Values are everywhere.
- Values are action guiding.

This supports our call for a broader view where values are seen across the perspective, but are also in the foreground as well as in the background, influencing the decisions that are made. There is still, however, a question about how values and ethics actually relate.

We would put it this way. Attention to values broadens the horizon, but values themselves sharpen the ethical view. For needs, wishes, preferences and so forth immediately give rise to ethical concerns, particularly in a context where they are being ignored either wholly or partly. Values, therefore, seem to lead to ethics, because there is a moral imperative not to ignore values in the same way that we cannot ignore facts. Facts tend to be value-laden. But if they are not, then they are *just* facts. Values, however, are never *just* values. Values, we might say, awaken ethical concerns. But they do more than this, because they also pull us back to the broader view of persons situated in numerous fields of history, culture, law, familial, social networks, and so forth. Our moral worlds are finely nuanced and interconnecting. In a sense, this takes us back to virtue ethics, where to flourish or do well as a human being is multifaceted. It requires all of our practical and intellectual skill and understanding. This is because the complex world in which we act is a world of other persons where values are everywhere and are ever-changing. The world of values, therefore, is also the world of political and social relationships (as well as ethics) in wider society. It is the world of citizenship, where we engage, not just as individuals but also as citizens. Again, this takes us back to the relevance of the Nuffield Council's Ethical Framework (Table 5.2), where Components 5 and 6 had to do with solidarity and personhood. We cannot escape the relevance of these notions.

Conclusions

We can now add to the conclusions about values:

- Values are wider than ethics.
- Values are everywhere.
- Values are action guiding.

But also,

- Values awaken ethical concerns.
- Values encourage a broader view.

Reasoning about values naturally leads us to ethical concerns, when we have to decide on the best course of action to take. But this, in turn, is related to the nature of our personhood as situated agents in an interconnecting world, where what is required is solidarity. The world of values, amidst many other things, is an ethical and political world. It is a world in which people engage as citizens.

The bigger picture, then, is to see ourselves as persons (potentially) with dementia in the context of a *polis* or state in which we act as citizens. As we shall see, this bigger picture emphasizes the extent to which we must see ourselves, including people with dementia, as the bearers of rights. Thinking about values, therefore, encourages thoughts about citizenship and about the nature of our participation in the *polis*. Values-based practice suggests the need for a focus on rights. But more of that later! For now, we can at least assert the following:

1. Dementia reflects our humanity.
2. Dementia highlights disability rights as much as any difficulties associated with disease.
3. VBP provides a way to tackle difficult situations in dementia care and to uphold the rights of the individual.

Key Points

- Awareness of values throws up ethical dilemmas.
- To decide which values must be given weight requires ethical consideration.
- Values awareness also helps to broaden the picture such that persons are seen as situated in contexts.

- Ethical judgements, therefore, involve applying theories, approaches, and frameworks which reflect particular concrete contexts and yet a multiplicity of perspectives.
- We make decisions by taking the broadest possible view of contexts and perspectives, concerning which our decision making must employ clear and coherent arguments and rational thought.
- Into this process we must bring a broad array of concerns, including facts, but also emotions, inclinations, stories, and values.
- Furthermore, the broader view, encouraged by attention to values, situates us as persons (with or without dementia) in a *polis* – a state – in which individuals have rights and duties as citizens, which are designed (ideally) to maintain and protect our values.

References

Beauchamp, T. L. and Childress, J. F. (2008). *Principles of Biomedical Ethics* (6th Edition). Oxford and New York: Oxford University Press.

Culley, H., Barber, R., Hope, A., and James, I. (2013). Therapeutic lying in dementia care. *Nursing Standard* **28**: 35–39.

Dresser, R. (1995). Dworkin on dementia: Elegant theory, questionable policy. *Hastings Center Report* **25**: 32–38.

Dworkin, R. (1993). *Life's Dominion: An Argument about Abortion and Euthanasia.* London: Harper Collins.

Fulford, K. W. M. (Bill), Peile, E., and Carroll, H. (2012). *Essential Values-Based Practice: Clinical Stories Linking Science with People.* Cambridge: Cambridge University Press.

Greener, H., Poole, M., Emmett, C. et al. (2012). Value judgements and conceptual tensions: Decision-making in relation to hospital discharge for people with dementia. *Clinical Ethics* **7**: 166–174.

Hughes, J. C. (2001). Views of the person with dementia. *Journal of Medical Ethics* **27**: 86–91.

(2011). *Thinking through Dementia.* Oxford: Oxford University Press.

(2013). Ethics in old age psychiatry. In T. Denning and A. Thomas, eds., *Oxford Textbook of Old Age Psychiatry* (2nd edition). Oxford: Oxford University Press, pp. 725–743.

Hughes, J. C. and Baldwin, C. (2006). *Ethical Issues in Dementia Care: Making Difficult Decisions.* London and Philadelphia: Jessica Kingsley.

Hughes, J. C., Beatty, A., and Shippen, J. (2014). Sexuality in dementia. In C. Foster, J. Herring, and I. Doron, eds., *The Law and Ethics of Dementia.* Oxford: Hart Publishers, pp. 227–238.

James, I. A., Wood-Mitchell, A., Waterworth, A. M., Mackenzie, L., and Cunningham, J. (2006). Lying to people with dementia: Developing ethical guidelines for care settings. *International Journal of Geriatric Psychiatry* **21**: 800–801.

Jaworska, A. (1999). Respecting the margins of agency: Alzheimer's patients and the capacity to value. *Philosophy and Public Affairs* **28**: 105–138.

Williamson, T. and Kirtley, A. (2016). *What Is Truth? An Inquiry about Truth, Lying, Different Realities and Beliefs in Dementia Care* (Review of Evidence and Report). London: Mental Health Foundation. Available via: www.mentalhealth.org.uk/publications/what-truth-inquiry-about-truth-and-lying-dementia-care (last accessed 26 December 2017).

Relationships – Values and Person-Centred Care

Topics covered in this chapter

- This chapter is about relationships and the many and various ways in which they affect the care of people living with dementia.
- This is seen in particular in VBP's emphasis on person-centred practice (or person-values-centred practice).
- Dementia poses unique tensions in relationships and in the practical implementation of person-centred practice.
- The importance of rights in addition to the processes of VBP is evident, but rights themselves embody values.
- Getting the correct balance between the views and values of the person living with dementia and his or her carer(s) is a central and crucial task for all concerned.

Take-away message for practice

People living with dementia may or may not be able to express their values, so judgements have to be made. But such judgements must take note of the views of those with whom they are in close caring relationships. Judgements about the nature of those relationships must also be made, with attention being paid to your own values and your relationships with all those involved.

Introduction

This chapter tests VBP to the limit. Dementia really stretches at least one key factor in VBP in order for it to 'work' for people with the condition. This factor is *person-centred practice*, but as the title indicates, this chapter focuses on relationships, for several reasons that will be explained. Although relationships *per se* don't exist as a separate category in VBP's ten key pointers to good process, the importance of relationships is clearly implicit in some, and fairly explicit in others, such as being multidisciplinary in approach and working in partnership. Reference to relationships will be made in the chapters which focus on these other pointers, but it is *person-centred practice* that provides the clearest way to explore the relevance of relationships to dementia.

There is perhaps no other major health condition where relationships are so important yet also as complex as they are in the field of dementia. VBP is of immense help in providing tools to focus on the values, and people, in those relationships. This chapter describes how paying attention to relationships is essential for the successful application of VBP in the care and support of people with dementia. A focus on relationships underpins both the premise of VBP – *mutual respect for differences of values* – and its point – *balanced decision making within a framework of shared values*. Yet at the same time the premise, process, and point of VBP must also be *rights compatible*; practitioners need to be aware of the legal frameworks that they are working within, the impact these may have on relationships, and how to support and inform others about these frameworks whenever necessary.

Relationships

The importance of positive relationships – intimate partnerships and marriages, family relationships, friendships, therapeutic relationships – in maintaining a person's positive mental health and assisting people to cope with and recover from periods of mental distress cannot be overestimated. An absence of relationships, or being involved in negative or abusive relationships, can contribute to or cause a mental health problem and also make it much harder to recover or cope with the problem. This applies just as much to people with dementia, and there is evidence to indicate that loneliness may be a significant factor in the onset and development of some dementias. As we shall see, however, a combination of the effects of dementia and their impact on the relationships that people with dementia commonly have make VBP and person-centred practice particularly relevant.

The concept of the therapeutic relationship is central to health care. It is widely recognised (and supported by evidence) that without rapport, trust, understanding, and good communication between a service user and a practitioner, it is extremely difficult to assess, diagnose, and provide treatments or other health interventions successfully (e.g. McCabe and Priebe, 2004). Although the term 'therapeutic relationship' is not so widely used in social care, the underlying principles are just as valid. Yet as this chapter will explore, focusing on the therapeutic relationship for people with dementia is insufficient, because in many situations it does not address the diverse and complex relationships that exist for a person with dementia as the condition progresses.

The concept of the therapeutic relationship has been severely tested in some areas of health care, most notably mental health. For a number of reasons many mental health service users have rejected biopsychosocial explanations for their emotional, psychological or mental experiences. Consequently, the therapeutic component of the relationship has also been rejected or treated with suspicion, especially where it has simply been used to persuade or coerce the person into accepting treatment.

Person-centred practice is a key pointer in VBP's 'good process' that aims to provide more understanding and a greater emphasis on the values of the service user, as well as others, to try and overcome some of these difficulties. Mutual respect for differences of values must be expressed through relationships between people with dementia, carers, and practitioners, and those relationships are central to balanced decision making within a framework of shared values.

Person-Centred Practice

In the jargon of VBP, person-centred practice is often referred to as person-*values*-centred care. This is evident on the web pages of The Collaborating Centre for Values-Based

Practice in Health and Social Care, based at St. Catherine's College, University of Oxford (https://valuesbasedpractice.org). As it suggests, person-values-centred practice combines the more commonly used notion of person-centred care with a focus on values. The importance of this is in situations that regularly occur where there are *problems of conflicting values* and *problems of mutual understanding* between, for example, the person with dementia and their carer(s), or between professionals and carers.

Person-values-centred practice is defined as:

> practice that focuses on the values of the patient while at the same time being aware of and reflecting the values of other people involved (clinicians, managers, family, carers[1], etc.): this is important in tackling two particular problems of person-centred care, problems of mutual understanding and problems of conflicting values
>
> (Definition accessed from the VBP website 26 December 2017: www2.warwick.ac.uk/fac/med/study/research/vbp/about/glossary/)

It is important to note that although person-values-centred practice gives a particular emphasis to the values of the service user – and this should always be the starting point for decisions and actions involving care and treatment – it does not say that they are the *only* point, or that they 'trump' the values of everyone else. This inclusive approach is crucial to VBP. (Henceforth, however, in keeping with *Essential Values-Based Practice* (Fulford et al., 2012) we shall only talk of person-centred practice, because, in our view, any notion of the person worth its salt must contain the idea of values: it is part of the situatedness of persons, and '[p]ersons are inevitably situated in a world of norms' (Hughes, 2011; p. 228).)

Hitherto VBP has focused on people with physical disorders and 'functional' mental illnesses, but not dementia. Fulford et al. (2012) includes examples of people with mental health problems, and *Model Values* (Mental Health Foundation, 2004) is entirely devoted to using VBP in mental health practice. So these provide a useful starting place for considering how person-centred practice might be applied in dementia care. Because mental health problems generally do not manifest themselves in physical ways, they are often harder to define and diagnose, and conflicts often arise between a service user and others about whether their experiences are a 'life' problem or a genuine mental disorder – there can be quite different understandings of the problem between those involved. Similarly, the early stages of dementia may not immediately appear to be symptoms of the condition, giving rise to different explanations, and different understandings of dementia may persist between people with dementia, carers, and practitioners even after it has been diagnosed.

The shift away from institutional mental health care towards care in the community, recognition in many parts of the mental health system of the imbalance in the relationship between professionals and service users (and carers), and the growing strength and influence of service user voices also brought a sharp focus onto differences in values in mental health care. Incorporating person-centred practice has therefore been very relevant in the provision of mental health care and treatment. The changes also signified a shift away from a disease model approach towards a disability model, though the shift was not as dramatic as for other disability groups. Although the voices of people with dementia have not been so noticeable, and institutional-type care in the form of care

---

[1] The quote differentiates families from carers. As previously indicated, this book uses the common definition of carer to mean anyone in an unpaid, informal caring role, which includes family and friends but not paid staff or volunteers working in a supportive or caring role.

homes is still common for many people with more severe dementia, the need to focus on the person, rather than just the dementia, has become more widely acknowledged by dementia practitioners, particularly given the limited evidence base for treatments and other interventions in dementia care.

The issue of rights is another similarity, as many jurisdictions have mental health and mental capacity (sometimes referred to as 'competency') legislation, which allows decisions to be made and action to be taken on behalf of a person with a mental health condition, including dementia, where the person lacks capacity to make the decision or refuses to give their consent. As already described in Chapter 2 these laws generally try to strike a balance between respecting a person's autonomy and protection from harm (or harm to others), as well as being compliant with wider human rights and equality legislation (e.g., the prohibition of detention without a proper legal process, not treating people unfairly based upon age or a physical or mental disability), which practitioners have to be mindful of in any case. When these come into play together with other rights, such as statutory entitlements to services, person-centred practice and relationships become considerably more complex.

Despite these similarities, there are significant differences between people with dementia and other mental health service users in terms of relationships and applying person-centred practice. Here are three of importance:

- Although some mental health problems can be severe and long term, none is as organic, progressive, and potentially terminal as dementia. The majority of people experience some form of recovery from an episode of mental illness or distress. Their values may change over time, but they continue to be able to express these themselves. As dementia progresses, it generally becomes harder and harder for the person to express the values that are important to them because of difficulties of cognition, memory, and communication. The person may also start expressing new or different values from those they had before the dementia developed, and it can be very difficult for others to know whether these are 'true' expressions of the person's values or solely symptoms of the dementia (or both). It is perfectly possible that a person's values can change over time, and given the long duration of a dementia illness, it may well be the case that for numerous reasons the person's values could change in this period.

- Mental health problems can be experienced at any time of life, but more serious episodes of psychosis or behaviours associated with personality disorders (arguably the main focus of specialist mental health services) most commonly appear among younger adults, who are less likely to have long-standing relationships or families separate from the family they were born into. Almost without exception, dementia is a condition that does not appear until late middle age and later life. People with dementia are therefore much more likely to have families and long-standing live-in partners. The values of a person with dementia may be the same as or well known to their partner or family – they are personal but often mutual values that exist in the relationship (although this may change, as previously indicated). Yet as this chapter goes on to describe, if partners, family members, or close friends need to express the values of the person with dementia because they are unable to do this themselves, it can be unclear if these really are the person's values (similar difficulties can arise where professionals or care staff do this on behalf of the person with dementia).

- Many people with dementia, especially those diagnosed early, live with the condition for many years. Mainstream medicine and health care are limited in what they can currently offer because of the lack of cures and universally effective treatments or interventions with a clear evidence base. Carers therefore provide much of the support to the individual in the early to mid-stages of the illness. The impairments associated with dementia may make it feel like caring for someone with a disability rather than a disease. Health and social care services become more involved as the dementia makes it more difficult for the person and carers to cope; this creates new relationships and can change the dynamics in existing ones, particularly when a person with dementia has to move away from their family and loved ones and into residential care. This is discussed in more detail later.

To illustrate some of these points, let's consider a vignette.

Vignette – Mr Lloyd (Part 1)

Mr Lloyd is 78 years old and lives with his wife, aged 76, in their own home. They have a daughter who lives nearby and visits twice a week. She has her own family with two small children. Mr and Mrs Lloyd also have a son who lives several hours' drive away and visits very infrequently. He is divorced and, whenever he does visit, he complains of his 'money problems', which often results in arguments with Mr Lloyd.

Six years ago, Mr Lloyd was diagnosed with Alzheimer's disease. He had become noticeably forgetful and had two minor car accidents. This was most unlike him. He had also gotten lost on several occasions when driving back from his social club, which he visited on a weekly basis on a route he had driven for years. After receiving his diagnosis, and because of these incidents, Mr Lloyd reluctantly agreed to give up his driving licence. However, he refused to talk about his cognitive difficulties or acknowledge he had Alzheimer's disease. Instead, he had elaborate explanations for any problems which involved the police, the effect of dental treatments he had years previously, and 'misunderstandings'.

For three years after being diagnosed the Lloyds coped well at home, but things became more difficult as the Alzheimer's progressed. Although Mr Lloyd liked to drink and smoke and these had always been in moderation, his behaviour after he had a drink was becoming more unpredictable, and Mrs Lloyd was getting very worried about him being a fire hazard because he left lit cigarettes balanced on ashtrays (he had a small room in the house where he smoked). His sleep pattern also became increasingly erratic, staying up late into the night or getting up at odd hours. This resulted in arguments between the two of them, with Mr Lloyd refusing to stop smoking or drinking. As time went by these arguments became worse, with Mr Lloyd shouting and threatening and Mrs Lloyd becoming increasingly scared. Although by this time Mr Lloyd was under the care of a consultant psychiatrist and was visited by a community psychiatric nurse (CPN) on a regular basis, he always tried to avoid talking to them, rarely acknowledged anything they had to say to him, and according to Mrs Lloyd said that 'the doctors just wanted to put him in a home'. As a result, practitioners focused their attention on offering advice and support to Mrs Lloyd. Their daughter sometimes tried to mediate between her parents, as she got on well with both of them, but could not resolve the situation. Both Mr and Mrs Lloyd were insistent that they didn't want paid care staff coming into their house.

A year and half ago, Mr Lloyd accidentally started a small fire, which resulted in an armchair being burnt and the fire brigade being called. As a result of this incident all the professionals involved urged the family to consider residential care for Mr Lloyd. Mrs Lloyd reluctantly admitted that she was finding it very difficult to cope, and her children agreed (the son suddenly seemed to take a particular interest in the situation). Mrs Lloyd and her daughter were absolutely adamant that they didn't want professionals telling him that he would be going to a care home because they believed he would be very resistant and distressed about the idea of a move like this. Instead, Mrs Lloyd and her daughter told Mr Lloyd that he was just going away temporarily to stay in a hotel while the fire damage was repaired and they did not want this story contradicted. Somewhat reluctantly the professionals agreed to this approach, and three months later Mr Lloyd moved into the Valhalla Care Home, seven miles from where he had lived, with the understanding that he was going there for a temporary stay.

Commentary

From the story so far, we can immediately see the problems of mutual understanding and conflicting values. How can person-centred practice help address the challenges and complexities both of focusing on the values of Mr Lloyd and of being aware and actively working with the values of Mr Lloyd's family, whilst at the same time upholding professional values?

- *Working with values in unconventional 'therapeutic' relationships.* On the surface at least, Mr Lloyd's values appear not to be consciously driven by an awareness of his Alzheimer's. He doesn't use it as a term to describe his situation, uses alternative explanations, and avoids contact with health care professionals. According to his family he would not be willing to move into a care home.

Person-centred practice points practitioners in the direction of acknowledging and perhaps having partially to work with the values Mr Lloyd expresses, rather than ignoring or rejecting them because they are 'wrong' or because he 'lacks insight'. Although some people with dementia may experience fluctuating realities with periods of lucidity as well as of confusion, once it is evident that an alternative reality is fixed and immovable, practitioners need to be more flexible and responsive in how they engage with a person. Rejecting or ignoring the different reality of a person with dementia is unlikely to help in building a relationship, denies practitioners the opportunity to find out more about what the person may be experiencing (is it an expression of an unmet need or an attempt to make sense of reality, for example?), and may cause distress or have other negative impacts on the person's self-esteem and sense of identity. Respecting and exploring what's important to Mr Lloyd, and what therefore might be guiding his actions (e.g. loss of independence and opportunities to socialize), provides a potential bridge into establishing trust and negotiating positive interventions that may help him.

However, it has to be acknowledged that the situation leading up to the move into the care home was born out of values of necessity and safety, and was not something that reflected Mr Lloyd's values. Moves into care homes where the person is not told the truth or does not agree but where the move is regarded as being in his or her best interests are quite common, yet clearly pose a test for person-centred practice. It demonstrates how torn people's values can become, such as Mrs Lloyd's: between wanting to look after her husband on the one hand, but fearful for her own safety (and his) on the other. For person-centred practice to have worked to enable Mr Lloyd to stay at home, it would have required greater alignment of values with Mr Lloyd's (who would have had, for example, to accept care staff into the house and be willing to take more risk) and the resources to operationalize those values. In the absence of this, the existing relationships of care could not be sustained.

- *Working with values in proxy relationships.* Mr Lloyd has long-standing family relationships (though not entirely straightforward ones). It is Mrs Lloyd in particular who is experiencing and having to deal with the effect of Mr Lloyd's Alzheimer's as a major, uninvited addition to their lives and their relationship. Although many people in Mrs Lloyd's position still primarily define themselves as 'wife', 'husband', 'partner', etc., it is also clear that they have had to assume the role of carer. This may significantly change the relationship they have with the person with dementia (rarely do people enter relationships knowing or desiring someone to become increasingly dependent upon them), and gender roles can play a significant factor in shaping this. It also means they become part of an 'extended' multidisciplinary care team. Unfortunately, as Mr Lloyd's condition deteriorates, his values (autonomy, 'doing what he wants to do') diverge from Mrs Lloyd's and her daughter's (personal safety, 'not having to worry all the time').

Person-centred practice emphasizes the importance of taking into account the values of carers, and in dementia care this is particularly important. Carers may share many of the values of the person with dementia or know them intimately and can be essential proxies and advocates for the person's values. Of course, they may have their own values which, as we shall see, can be in conflict with the person with dementia, or may become confused with the values of the person with dementia. Quality-of-life studies show that carers may struggle at times to separate their own experiences when asked about the quality of life of the person with dementia they care for (Beer et al., 2010; Williamson, 2010).

Carers are also not employed as members of Mr Lloyd's care team and are therefore not bound by the team's organizational or professional values. Unlike dementia practitioners, this may be the first time they have ever encountered dementia, and there is a chance that they will do whatever works best on a day-to-day, practical, and emotional level to maintain positive family relationships and wellbeing for both themselves and Mr Lloyd. Evidence indicates that information, education, and support from practitioners and other carers can be extremely helpful in enabling carers to cope and reduce stress (La Fontaine et al., 2013).

• *Working with values in compromised relationships.* Practitioners involved in Mr Lloyd's care were largely reliant upon the relationship they had with Mrs Lloyd and her daughter in order to get information about Mr Lloyd's health and how his Alzheimer's was affecting him. Although they were successful in convincing the family that Mr Lloyd could no longer be cared for safely at home, the nature of the relationship they had with the family, and the reliance on them to negotiate the move to the care home, meant they had to 'go along' with the story they told Mr Lloyd about the move.

Person-centred practice points to a default position whereby practitioners should always try and involve carers in how care is planned and delivered to people with dementia, especially when they are living in their own home. Carers can be an essential and sometimes the only source of reliable information about how dementia is affecting someone. They are caring for the person on a daily basis and, as with Mr Lloyd, are of fundamental importance in negotiating a significant change in his or her life. But their values as carers are born out of personal experience and necessity, not choice of profession, so values diversity and compromise may well have to be applied in negotiating and supporting them, as much as it is with the person with dementia. Practitioners may have felt uncomfortable about the story told to Mr Lloyd about the move into the care home and may have had ethical or moral objections to apparent collusion with what appears to be a lie. However, these values had to be put to one side for practical reasons, but also in order to maintain the crucial relationship with the family as carers and as a way of knowing what was happening with Mr Lloyd.

Of course, there may be particular reasons why it is problematic working with carers, especially where there is suspicion, hostility, or fundamental disagreements. Practitioners should be aware of the values created for some carers by the stigma and fear that dementia can generate through the media, as well as the power that professionals are perceived to have, together sometimes with their own negative experiences of health and social care. If the person with dementia has expressed specific requests or has capacity and makes it clear they do not want a particular family member involved in discussions about their care, then their wishes should be respected. However, a person's awareness of the effects of their dementia may deteriorate more rapidly than their ability to communicate – they may say things are fine when in fact they are experiencing a lot of difficulties. Carers are likely to carry this knowledge, so if the carer is not present in a clinical consultation or care planning meeting, it is important that practitioners find ways of checking out how things are without going behind the back of the person with dementia. Where there are difficulties in having a relationship with carers, these need to be acknowledged and the reasons recorded – it could be that a practitioner from another team, or voluntary sector organization, or an advocate might mediate a relationship.

- *Pressure of time, resources, and context.* Applying person-centred practice may appear to be yet another task to be carried out, when a variety of factors militate against this. The need to 'do something' about Mr Lloyd's situation as things get more difficult at home appears to be the priority, rather than (what may seem to be) an unnecessary discussion about values. But the discussion about what needs to be done can and should involve talk about values, because this is much more likely to result in better decisions being made and actions taken. A clinical consultation, assessment, care planning meeting, best-interests meeting, or discussion with the family – or a combination of these – all provide opportunities to gain awareness and knowledge of the different values in play and to record them.
- *Rights, values, and relationships (Part 1).*

The situation prior to Mr Lloyd's move into the care home and the move itself also raise a number of issues about the conflicting rights of those involved. Under the MCA, Mr Lloyd has the right to make his own decisions, even if these are unwise ones, but if he lacks capacity, then decisions can be made on his behalf in his best interests. Mr Lloyd wants to stay at home, but issues of safety and the risk posed by Mr Lloyd both to himself and to Mrs Lloyd also have to be taken into account. If Mr Lloyd lacks capacity to make decisions about living at home safely and his actions are caused by his dementia, then from a safeguarding point of view it might be argued that both he and Mrs Lloyd have a right to protection from possible harm – either through increasing the support and supervision Mr Lloyd gets at home or through the move into the care home. However, in the UK, publicly funded social care at home or in a care home is not a universal right but is dependent upon severity of need and a person's financial circumstances (except in Scotland where it is currently free). A right to services for some is a question of choice and an expense for others. If Mr Lloyd were entitled to publicly funded social care, his right to be supported at home might come under pressure from social services because of resource issues. A move into a care home, rightly or wrongly, might be presented as the only safe way of delivering his right to social care. Equally, there can be times when the social care budget means that people are encouraged to stay at home past the stage at which the carer can really manage. Finally, even if Mr Lloyd were deemed to have capacity, his diagnosis of dementia and the worry about safety could lead to him being detained under mental health legislation for assessment, ensuring (in theory) Mr Lloyd's right to an assessment of his health, though it is unlikely that he would experience compulsory assessment in that way. In all of these situations, relationships are woven into rights. For Mr Lloyd to exercise his rights, or for him and Mrs Lloyd to be safe, others may have to intervene, altering relationships because actions taken may be based on new or different values from those expressed previously.

Issues of confidentiality also arise and carry practical and legal concerns. These are discussed in more detail in Chapter 7, but it is worth making some comments in relation to confidentiality and Mr Lloyd. First, it is possible (though unlikely) that Mr Lloyd may have agreed with members of his family that they could be included in discussions about him, even in his absence. As we shall discuss in Chapter 9, an early diagnosis of dementia enables a discussion to take place with the person about who else can be included in discussions about them – and it is important to record this. Where a person has not given their consent and they lack capacity to make this decision, confidential information can still be shared, providing it is in their best interests. Although, as we have seen in Chapter 4, the MCA's primary focus is on the individual who may or may not have capacity to make a decision, the law also recognizes the importance of others, including carers, in helping with the assessment of capacity and making best-interests decisions, recognizing the knowledge and values that others bring. Situations where a person does have capacity and refuses consent are more challenging – but this should be used to start a conversation about the importance of involving family and the difficulties caused, especially over time, if they are excluded.

As circumstances change, so, too, can the values and relationships that people with dementia have. Matters can be further illustrated by continuing with Mr Lloyd's story.

Vignette – Mr Lloyd (Part 2)

Initially Mr Lloyd settled into the care home well, saying he was happy to be there, and was visited regularly by Mrs Lloyd and their daughter. However, as time went by Mrs Lloyd found the visits increasingly difficult because her husband started asking when he would be going home. He sometimes became upset or angry with her when she was vague in her reply. She told both her daughter and the care home staff that she wasn't going to visit so often and felt she had done the wrong thing by moving Mr Lloyd into the care home. Mr Lloyd also started saying that a young member of the care staff was his daughter, not recognizing his real daughter when she visited, and he insisted on introducing the care home worker to her as his real daughter. His daughter found this very upsetting and had several arguments with the staff about how they should handle this. Mr Lloyd's son only visited him once and said it was the best place for him and that he was going to encourage Mrs Lloyd to sell their house and move into something smaller. This upset the rest of the family, and Mr Lloyd, meanwhile, became more physically agitated and demanding about going home, repeatedly talking about staff as 'warders' and saying he had 'done his time'. When Mrs Lloyd heard about this on one of her visits, she said it must be to do with him remembering being in the army and serving a short period of time in a military prison. At times, however, he still enjoyed visits from his family even when he struggled to recognize them.

Mr Lloyd's behaviour became increasingly difficult to manage, and staff at the care home came to the view that he clearly did not have capacity to agree to stay at the home. The care home manager was aware that this could mean Mr Lloyd's human rights were being violated if he needed to stay in the home under close supervision, because he was being deprived of his liberty without any legal safeguards. Under the MCA, several assessments were carried out, including of his capacity to consent to being in the home. There was also a best-interests assessment to determine whether he needed to be cared for in the home. Mrs Lloyd and her daughter were involved in these discussions. Subsequently an application from the care home for Deprivation of Liberty Safeguards (DoLS) was approved by the local authority, meaning that Mr Lloyd at least had some protective rights while he was staying in the home.

Commentary

The move into the care home had addressed one set of important concerns and values but in doing so had generated a new set of values, shown by the new relationships and dynamics that developed.

- *Changing relationships – shifting values.* Mr Lloyd's move into the care home has resulted in new relationships being formed and changes in existing ones, all giving rise to more challenges around conflicting values and problems of mutual understanding. His relationship with his family has changed, and their values have been affected by the move. Relationships within the family have also changed. Different family members consider different things to be important, and their relationships with care home staff can generate tensions. The move has brought into greater focus the value Mr Lloyd places on independence and his reluctance to be confined, as well as perhaps his need for comfort and familiarity. It also appears that he has 'time shifted' to an earlier period in his life – a common occurrence for people with dementia – when his daughter, for instance, was younger and to a period when he was a prisoner.

Person-centred practice emphasizes the need for all these values to be understood and taken into account. While there is a need at a practical day-to-day level to manage Mr Lloyd's behaviour, it is crucial that time is set aside to discuss the different values being expressed and be open about the conflicts these give rise to; VBP emphasizes the importance of a process to enable this to happen. Practitioners with experience in dementia may need to advise and support care home staff about the reasons for Mr Lloyd's behaviour. As when he was living in his own home, staff will need at least to acknowledge that the different reality he is experiencing and the values thereby expressed are very real to him and a cause of distress. As touched on in Chapter 5, a range of possible interventions can be considered and applied (Williamson and Kirtley, 2016).

While the focus of practitioners must be on Mr Lloyd, it is also crucial that time and consideration are given to his family. Unlike Mr Lloyd, other members of the family are not cognitively impaired and, therefore, through talking with them about Mr Lloyd and the effects of his dementia, it may be possible to help them come to terms with the situation. Although Mr Lloyd may no longer recognize his daughter and at times expresses anger towards his wife, he still seems to appreciate their visits and, therefore, it is important to encourage them to keep coming but provide them with support if the visits are difficult. Staff can make time to meet regularly with the family and to explain the effects of the dementia and the consequences for the values Mr Lloyd expresses. It may be possible to work with the changes brought about by the dementia to improve his wellbeing and that of the family, which is an important value in its own right and one embedded in law in England through the Care Act 2014. It may also be helpful for Mr Lloyd's family to understand his dementia in terms of a disability, as well as a disease, and to support him it will be easier for others to adapt than to change his behaviour or his perception of the world.

However, family members may not feel comfortable with strategies used by staff, especially if they go against their own values and moral codes (e.g., to do with truth-telling) or those of the person with dementia. Similarly, being expected to ignore or even deny a long-standing relationship or identity (husband/wife, father/daughter, in the Lloyds' case) may be very upsetting and take some time to come to terms with. Acknowledging the feelings of the family, especially Mrs Lloyd's apparent sense of guilt and the daughter's sense of rejection, and giving them support are therefore important things for staff to do. It may also be helpful for Mrs Lloyd and her daughter to meet other relatives of people living in the home, perhaps to become more involved in the life of the home in general, or to derive support from a dementia carers group if one exists locally.

- *Rights, values, and relationships (Part 2).* The need for the DoLS and the sense that Mr Lloyd's son has ulterior motives about the move into the care home, connected with his financial situation, generates an additional focus on Mr Lloyd's rights under the law. DoLS are a complicated legal framework,[2] and criticisms of them may lead to reform, but the important point here is that in principle they provide legal safeguards for the need to care for Mr Lloyd in the home. This may provide some reassurance to Mrs Lloyd. The challenge posed by the son points to the importance of practitioners being aware of the legal framework governing situations for people who lack capacity to make their own decisions. The MCA provides ways for people to express their wishes, feelings, values, and beliefs in advance through oral or written statements, which should be taken into account in best-interests decisions, advance decisions to refuse treatment (which can be legally binding), and a process for authorizing others to make decisions on a person's behalf, known as Lasting Powers of Attorney (LPAs).[3] LPAs can authorize someone (usually trusted family members) to make best-interests decisions about a person's health, care, and welfare and about their property and financial affairs. Although it might have been difficult to get Mr Lloyd to make an LPA when he still had capacity, it could have helped clarify who made decisions about the family home. Even a simple statement by Mr Lloyd of his wishes, values, and beliefs would have been useful, or a brief life story[4] (biography) would have been helpful, especially for care home staff who don't know him very well.

Nevertheless, values contained in legal rights can be daunting and complicated – entitlement to publicly funded social care (including residential care) is often determined by severity of need and by a person's financial situation, unlike jurisdictions that provide free health care at the point of need. Furthermore, although laws like the MCA should be compliant with human rights legislation, it is not currently clear if this is the case with the United Nations Convention on the Rights of Persons with Disabilities (which can apply to people with dementia). Person-centred practice needs to involve an understanding of these legal frameworks and the values inherent in them, and needs to be explained to people in a helpful and informative way.

---

[2] Good, clear information about DoLS is available from the British Medical Association (BMA), the Royal College of Psychiatrists, and the Social Care Institute for Excellence (SCIE).

[3] For more information on these, see the *Mental Capacity Act Code of Practice.*

[4] Creating and having access to a person's life story is increasingly common in the dementia field as it helps maintain a focus on the person, not just the dementia, and can help guide decisions about care and treatment. Life story work is recognized as having an evidence base by the National Institute for Health and Care Excellence. For more information see www.lifestorynetwork.org.uk.

Reflection points

Although Mr Lloyd's scenario is fairly typical in terms of family structure and relationships, together with the responses from health and social care, it is important to point out some of the significant variations in relationships and values that bring other values into play. Here are some examples.

- *Non-disclosure of diagnosis.* For a variety of reasons people are sometimes not told about their dementia diagnosis. In Mr Lloyd's case this may not have made any difference, but if someone isn't told the reasons why their memory, cognition, or ability to communicate is causing problems, it potentially creates difficult situations for family members, friends, and practitioners in terms of how they relate to the person with dementia. Non-disclosure of diagnosis may occur because it's believed that it would cause unnecessary distress, but this has to be carefully weighed against the difficulties caused by dementia and not know- ing the reasons why. A fiction or avoidance has to be used by those caring for the person, which may run contrary to the values of carers and practitioners. Would there have been any advantage in not telling Mr Lloyd his diagnosis? This is explored more in Chapter 10.
- *Diverse family structures.* Family structures are increasingly diverse as a result of divorce, separation, second marriages, stepchildren, and so on. These family struc- tures may have difficult dynamics, irrespective of a person's dementia, bringing in new and additional values affecting a situation.
- *More than one person with dementia, more than one carer.* Increased life expectancy and an increase in people being diagnosed early may mean that people from two gen- erations within a family have dementia. Both people in a partnership or marriage may have dementia. Carers may also therefore be needing care, which might be because of dementia, but can be because of other conditions too (e.g. advanced arthritis or cancer).
- *Early-onset dementia.* It is now estimated that there are over 40,000 people under the age of 65 in the UK who have early-onset dementia. This means that there are growing numbers of people who are still in employment who are diagnosed with dementia but may perhaps have young families and a mortgage to pay. The values of employ- ers and financial institutions might therefore become important factors in decisions about care and treatment.
- *People with dementia from seldom-heard groups.* Consider the situation if Mr Lloyd were gay, transgender, or Black, Asian, or from another minority ethnic group. Services need to be inclusive and culturally competent, but the effects of dementia may have other sig- nificant consequences for those caring for the person. Anxieties about heteronormativity relating to an earlier phase in a person's life may become quite pronounced, especially in a care setting where the person is with people they don't know. Someone may revert to speaking in the language from their country of origin; other family members and practi- tioners may not be familiar with the language and struggle to communicate with the per- son. The person may also start behaving in a way or expressing wishes that run contrary to their faith or beliefs (such as eating non-kosher or non-halal meat). Should their 'new' values be accepted? Whereas practitioners may be more willing to respond positively to these new values, family members may find such changes hard to tolerate.
- *Attitudes of staff.* Care staff may object to being misidentified (e.g., as Mr Lloyd's daugh- ter). They may view it as unethical or feel uncomfortable with the fiction they have become part of, especially in situations where they are seen by the person with dementia in a negative role, such as prison guard. The person with dementia may also have time- shifted to when they were young, and care staff may become the object of unwanted attention (e.g., the person with dementia might become excessively flirtatious and phys- ically or sexually inappropriate). This can cross boundaries into the personal values of staff, and if no acknowledgement or discussion takes place with colleagues, staff may start avoiding, ignoring, mocking, teasing, or abusing the person in more serious ways.

The added complexity these variables create may at first seem mind-boggling in terms of awareness, knowledge, reasoning, and respect for differences of values and balanced decision making, especially when also endeavouring to be rights-compatible in one's practice. But these are long-standing challenges in the field of dementia, and in many respects VBP is ideally suited to providing a process to find solutions. Although testing for person-centred practice, they are not insurmountable, and it is worth considering at this point how VBP complements and potentially enhances some well-established approaches in dementia care.

Tom Kitwood and Person-Centred Care

It is important to acknowledge also how VBP links with other 'person-centred' approaches in dementia care. The work of Tom Kitwood, whom we have mentioned in earlier chapters, has been central to the development of the concepts of 'personhood' and 'person-centred care' in dementia practice (Kitwood, 1997). Commonplace in much dementia practice today, Kitwood's work was crucial in challenging what he saw as an excessive medicalization of dementia, at the expense of social and psychological factors, which removed a sense of the person and could easily result in very poor or even abusive practice, a process he described as 'malignant social psychology' (Kitwood, 1997: 45–49).

Central to Kitwood's thinking was the notion that the person retained a sense of self, no matter how severe the dementia had become, and that 'caregivers' (Kitwood's term) should never lose sight of this, nor of the components that make up the self. Factors such as self-esteem, agency, confidence, and hope are fundamental to a sense of self, or 'personhood'; supporting and nurturing these should be central to dementia care practice.

Kitwood didn't explicitly write about values, but it is not difficult to draw parallels with VBP and add values to the components that are central to personhood. In this sense, there is a natural affinity between Kitwood's *person-centred care* and VBP's *person-centred practice*. Kitwood wrote less explicitly about relationships and did not focus that much on differences between family carers and practitioners. There is no doubt, however, that he saw relationships as central to care giving and care practice:

> To see personhood in relational terms is, I suggest, essential if we are to understand dementia.
>
> (Kitwood, 1997: 12)

> It is clear that caregiving, far from being something merely done 'to' or 'for' a needy person, is a truly cooperative and reciprocal engagement.
>
> (Baldwin and Capstick, 2007: 219–220)

Kitwood's work has been taken forward and developed. For instance, Dawn Brooker (2007) has characterized person-centred care by the acronym VIPS, which focuses on Valuing people, Individual's needs, Perspective of people with dementia, and Supportive psychology. VBP and person-centred care are therefore, broadly speaking, complementary to each other, and Kitwood's work points to how VBP can be 'customized' for dementia.

Dementia Care Models Involving Carers

More recently, however, the concept of person-centred care has been challenged and arguably enhanced in the field of dementia by giving greater acknowledgement to the relationships a person with dementia has, both with carers and practitioners. Greater awareness of these relationships, especially with carers, enhances our understanding of person-centred practice.

It has been said that living with dementia involves two sides of a coin – the person with dementia on one side and their carer(s)[5] on the other. Two-thirds of people with dementia in the UK live in their own homes in the community. It is estimated that there are 670,000 carers of people with dementia in the UK (the majority of whom are women) providing care worth £11 billion a year (Alzheimer's Society, 2014).

With the exception of professionals, up until fairly recently carers have been the dominant voice in speaking about dementia, particularly within voluntary (not-for-profit) dementia organizations such as the Alzheimer's Societies in the UK and elsewhere. This is understandable given that dementia has tended to be diagnosed late in its progression at a point when it becomes harder for the person to express their views independently, or to express them at all. The term 'service user' has often been seen by carers to incorporate *their* experience as well as that of the person with dementia, describing their role as proxy for the person with dementia. Many carers therefore consider that they, in effect, become the voice of the person living with dementia, and explicitly or implicitly they express the person's values as the dementia progresses. Take this (moving) quote from a carer speaking of her partner who is in the later stages of dementia (emphasis added):

> As the disease progresses and avenues of opportunity become cul-de-sacs, so his ability to meaningfully participate in the decision-making process in his life declines. I find my role even more essential to his continued well-being: fighting his corner to ensure dignity and comfort; calming his irrational fears; *maintaining the core values in his life* in these last months or years and preparing to do so at the end of his life.
>
> (Berkeley and Berkeley, 2014: 511)

Accordingly, forming a therapeutic relationship with the person with dementia is likely to involve forming a meaningful, if not therapeutic, relationship with their carer(s). A binary relationship becomes (at least) a triadic relationship. Acknowledging and working with this potential has enormous benefits, and a framework known as the 'triangle of care' has been developed in the UK to reflect the involvement of carers (Worthington et al., 2013).

Another important contribution has come from the work of Professor Mike Nolan and others, who have coined the phrase *relationship-centred care* (Nolan et al., 2001; Nolan et al., 2004). This enlarges the focus of person-centred care to consider both family relationships and friendships the person with dementia has, as well as relational practice: that is, the relationships between practitioners. Relationship-centred care emphasizes that good care must take into account these relationships (and, by implication, the values embedded in these relationships), and although not explicitly connected with it, complements and reinforces VBP.

Yet focusing on relationships also poses a significant challenge for practitioners trying to apply the concept of person-centred practice. Focusing on the values of the person with dementia may well involve having those values reported via the carer. Situations not previously encountered by the person living with dementia may arise where it seems

---

[5] This metaphor was frequently used, for example, in talks given by the late prominent UKPeter Ashley, although there is no specific reference for the metaphor.

essential to know their values but they are unable to express them, or where carers insist they – on behalf of the person – are best placed to express their values. A possible move into residential care and end-of-life decisions are two obvious examples. Where practitioners (or carers) are unsure of the person's values, where the person or carer is expressing values that are inconsistent with what had previously been said, or in a small number of cases where there are suspicions that the carer may have unscrupulous motives, person-centred practice looks like it becomes a potential minefield.[6]

Of course, it is also important to acknowledge that from the perspective of the person living with dementia and their carers, person-centred practice must be applied consistently and authentically by practitioners. The focus that is given to the values of the person with dementia and their carers may also be reciprocated when practitioners have their own values scrutinized by those they are caring for. There is considerable evidence from people with dementia and carers that the experience of assessment, diagnosis, and professional care has sometimes been very negative and unhelpful: carers have frequently been excluded from the process (often on the grounds of patient confidentiality), which seems unacceptable (Nuffield Council on Bioethics, 2009: 44–45), albeit where carers have been involved this has been experienced very positively (Williamson 2008; Newbronner et al., 2013).

However, it is also important to point out that there are a significant number of people with dementia who live alone. In 2010, 49 per cent of people aged 75 years and over in the UK lived alone (Office for National Statistics, 2010), so there is a high probability that many of these have dementia, although accurate data are hard to come by. Again, the majority are women because they have a greater life expectancy than men.

The position of carers in dementia care is well recognized and brings both benefits and challenges to the provision of care and treatment. In many situations, they come with their own values and the values of the person with dementia, which can be of enormous help to practitioners. These values can include the view that the carer is the mouthpiece of the person with dementia who can no longer express their own view. This may be true, but can sometimes reflect the carer assuming this role and taking over, perhaps because it takes longer for the person with dementia to think and answer questions. Practitioners need to be aware of this and steer conversations back to the person with dementia as much as possible, giving them time and support to participate in a discussion. If a carer really does need to be the spokesperson for the person with dementia, it is crucial that practitioners ascertain as far as possible whether the carer is expressing the genuine values of the person or whether these have been filtered, altered, or replaced by the carer's values.

The potential for problems of mutual understanding and conflicting values can be magnified in dementia care, compared to care in other situations where the person with the condition can express their wishes and feelings, beliefs, and values directly to practitioners. This reminds us that important though carers are, they are (usually) not the ones with dementia; person-centred practice emphasizes that the values of the person with dementia must be the key (but not the only) determinants for all actions by practitioners.

---

[6] However, a review of the literature looking at different types of 'centredness', e.g., person-centred, family-centred, relationship-centred care, and so forth, demonstrated that all of these different approaches actually shared the same central features and, in particular, person-centred care did not ignore relationships, and relationship-centred care did not ignore personhood (Hughes et al., 2008): 'The unifying themes of centredness, … reflect a movement in favour of increasing the social, psychological, cultural and ethical sensitivity of our human encounters'.

Conclusion

Relationships are ubiquitous and fundamental to people's lives (including when they are absent), and this applies just as much to people with dementia. Values are expressed through relationships and are the focus of person-centred practice.

Dementia care frequently involves complicated situations because of relationships, but the solutions offered by VBP are deceptively simple. The solutions require ongoing application of VBP's key practice skills: awareness and knowledge of the different values in play, reasoning to explore them, and clear communication, as well as empathy and acknowledgement of the emotions they invoke for all concerned. But the focus of VBP is on good process to discern values, not an assertion of whose values (and therefore solutions) are right and whose are wrong. The values involved in each situation will be different, reflecting the uniqueness of the individuals involved. Person-centred practice takes this into account, but as later chapters will describe, does not negate the facts in any given situation or the need to ensure decisions and actions are compatible with a framework of rights.

What should also be apparent throughout this chapter is that the three principles of our Manifesto remain salient:

- *Dementia as humanity.* The ways in which we, as persons, are embedded in our relationships – and how this at one and the same time both enhances and complicates our lives – are central to our humanity and to our lives with or without dementia, but are even more crucial where people are living with dementia.
- *Dementia as disease and disability.* Dementia as a disease can inhibit communication, but the perspective of disability rights makes us recognize that we, as individuals and as societies, must do our utmost to maintain the person's standing *as a person*.
- *VBP for dementia plus rights.* Whilst person-centred care is central to dementia care, the VBP approach enhances this perspective and is helpful to it. And especially when rights are brought into the frame, it is not solely the person's standing *as a person* but also his or her standing *as an active citizen* that is at issue. People with dementia must not be excluded from conversations about them. Relationships, therefore, are key.

Respecting differences in values and making balanced decisions within a framework of shared values can often be particularly challenging in dementia care because of relationships and difficulties in knowing the values of the person with dementia. But frequently there are sources that a practitioner can find to help with this:

- Expressions of values made in advance
- The knowledge carers have of a person's values
- Evidence from people with dementia (and carers) in testimonies, research, and policy statements drawn from people with dementia (referred to in Chapter 4)
- Other evidence about the needs and values of people with dementia when, for a variety of reasons such as cultural differences, less is known about what is important to them
- Values expressed in legal frameworks (which should be consistent with professional codes of practice, organizational values, etc.)
- Continuing awareness of contemporaneous values expressed by the person, even where they are not consistent with pre-morbid values.

Although these do not always provide answers and dilemmas still arise, using person-centred practice to explore values – of individuals through their relationships – provides a key element in VBP's emphasis on good process to support decisions and actions in dementia care. Of course, this takes time, places pressure on resources, and the urgency of a situation may militate against it. But rushing into attempts to find solutions without focusing on this process can easily backfire and cause more difficulties than it solves. Person-centred practice puts the spotlight on the values of the person with dementia, but it is not fixed; by shining a light on the values of carers and practitioners too, taking into account other, complementary approaches in dementia care, and ensuring such care remains within a rights-based framework, the chances of good, inclusive, decision making are greatly enhanced.

Key Points

- Dementia tests VBP to its limits because of dementia's progressive and terminal nature, the limited evidence base for treatments and other interventions for dementia, and typically the intimate and long-standing involvement of family and friends.
- The importance of human relationships involving people with dementia is central to this Manifesto – whether these are therapeutic (in the professional sense), caring, supportive, or loving. With only a limited evidence base for treatments and other interventions for dementia, the care and support for people with dementia must focus on and use the language of relationships as much as 'treatments' or 'interventions'.
- Values-based practice emphasizes the importance of the service user being the first source of information on values in any situation. However, this can be complicated in dementia care because of the effects of dementia and the involvement of people with close, long-standing relationships to the person – loved ones, extended family, and friends.
- While this Manifesto asserts that the person with dementia, and their values, must continue to be at the centre of their care, person-centred practice acknowledges that the provision of care must take into account carers and their values, as well as the values of practitioners.
- Numerous factors can complicate relationships in dementia care, not least of which is the difficulty of knowing the values of the person with dementia. Person-centred practice is demanding because it requires effort to ascertain these values, but there are sources of information that practitioners can go to. Simply reverting to solutions that may have worked in other situations, or ignoring all the values in play, is unlikely to provide lasting solutions, and may make matters worse.
- VBP and person-centred practice does not necessarily impose a new approach in dementia care at the expense of other approaches, but rather complements and enhances existing models that practitioners may already be familiar with. Person-centred practice can be incorporated into existing clinical and care processes, and values can be recorded alongside other aspects of a person's care.
- Despite the additional challenges that dementia can pose, person-centred practice provides a way of ensuring that all the values people have and their

relationships can be taken into account, and as far as possible, the pressure of resources, time, and context should not be used as an excuse to reject it. Mutual respect for differences of values and balanced decision making within a framework of shared values require person-centred practice as a key component.

- Person-centred practice must be compatible with a rights-based framework, and practitioners need to be aware of this. This Manifesto raises the bar of VBP with its emphasis on rights, but the values (and processes) described in legal frameworks should both help and enhance VBP in dementia care.

References

Alzheimer's Society. (2014). *Dementia 2014 Report Statistics*. Available via: www.alzheimers.org.uk/site/scripts/documents_info.php?documentID=341 (last accessed 26 December 2017).

Baldwin, C., and Capstick, A. (2007). *Tom Kitwood on Dementia: A Reader and Critical Commentary*. Maidenhead, Berkshire and New York: McGraw Hill, Open University Press.

Berkeley, S., and Berkeley, R. (2014). Lewy body disease: A carer's perspective. In C. Foster, J. Herring and I. Doron, eds., *The Law and Ethics of Dementia*. Oxford: Hart Publishers; pp. 509–11.

Beer, C., Flicker, L., Horner, B. et al. (2010). Factors associated with self and informant ratings of the quality of life of people with dementia living in care facilities: A cross sectional study. *PLoS ONE* 5(12): e15621. doi:10.1371/journal.pone.0015621

Brooker, D. (2007). *Person Centred Dementia Care: Making Services Better*. London: Jessica Kingsley.

Fulford, K.W.M. (Bill), Peile, E., and Carroll, H. (2012). *Essential Values-Based Practice: Clinical Stories Linking Science with People*. Cambridge: Cambridge University Press.

Hughes, J. C. (2011). *Thinking through Dementia*. Oxford: Oxford University Press.

Hughes, J. C., Bamford, C., and May, C. (2008). Types of centredness in health care: Themes and concepts. *Medicine, Health Care and Philosophy* 11, 455–63.

Kitwood, T. (1997). *Dementia Reconsidered*. Buckingham and Philadelphia: Open University Press.

La Fontaine, J., Jutlla, K., Read, K., Brooker, D., and Evans, S. (2013). *The Experiences, Needs and Outcomes for Carers of People with Dementia: Literature Review*. London: Royal Surgical Aid Society. Available via: www.thersas.org.uk/ (last accessed 23 December 2017).

McCabe, R., and Priebe, S. (2004). The therapeutic relationship in the treatment of severe mental illness: A review of methods and findings. *International Journal of Social Psychiatry* 50, 115–28.

Mental Health Foundation. (2009). *Model Values? Race, Values and Models in Mental Health*. London: Mental Health Foundation. Available via: www.mentalhealth.org.uk/sites/default/files/model_values.pdf (last accessed 23 December 2017).

Newbronner, L., Chamberlain, R., Borthwick, R., Baxter, M., and Glendinning, C. (2013). *A Road Less Rocky – Supporting Carers of People with Dementia*. London: Carers Trust. Available via: https://professionals.carers.org/sites/default/files/dementia_report_road_less_rocky_final_0.pdf (last accessed 26 December 2017).

Nolan, M., Keady, J., and Aveyard, B. (2001). Relationship-centred care is the next logical step. *British Journal of Nursing* 10: 757.

Nolan, M. R., Davies, S., Brown, J., Keady, J., and Nolan, J. (2004). Beyond person-centred care: A new vision for gerontological nursing. *Journal of Clinical Nursing* 13: 45–53.

Nuffield Council on Bioethics. (2009). *Dementia: Ethical Issues*. London: Nuffield Council on Bioethics. Available via: http://

nuffieldbioethics.org/project/dementia (last accessed 26 December 2017).

Office for National Statistics (2010). *General Lifestyle Survey Overview Report 2010*. Available via: www.ons.gov.uk/ons/rel/ghs/general-lifestyle-survey/2010/index.html (last accessed 26 December 2017).

Williamson, T. (2008). *Dementia: Out of the Shadows*. London: Alzheimer's Society. Available via: www.alzheimers.org.uk/download/downloads/id/876/my_name_is_not_dementia_people_with_dementia_discuss_quality_of_life_indicators.pdf (last accessed 26 December 2017).

(2010). *My Name Is Not Dementia: People with Dementia Discuss Quality of Life Indicators*. London: Alzheimer's Society. Available via: www.alzheimers.org.uk/download/downloads/id/876/my_name_is_not_dementia_people_with_dementia_discuss_quality_of_life_indicators.pdf (last accessed 23 December 2017).

Williamson, T., and Kirtley, A. (2016). *What Is Truth? An Inquiry about Truth, Lying, Different Realities and Beliefs in Dementia Care* (Review of Evidence and Report). London: Mental Health Foundation. Available via: www.mentalhealth.org.uk/publications/what-truth-inquiry-about-truth-and-lying-dementia-care (last accessed 26 December 2017).

Worthington, A., Rooney, P., and Hannan, R. (2013). *The Triangle of Care – Carers Included: A Guide to Best Practice in Mental Health Care in England*, 2nd edn. London: Carers Trust.

Working Together

Topics covered in this chapter
- This chapter is about working together in multidisciplinary teams (MDTs).
- In such teams, values will often be shared, but are nevertheless at play and should be recognized.
- This is partly because values within teams may sometimes conflict, in which case it is important to recognize differences in values (i.e. dissensus).
- Confidentiality is an important component of teamworking in health and social care.
- Between different cultures it is possible to see both shared and divergent values.

Take-away message for practice

MDTs can be thought of as groups that exist to explore and manifest values, to work with them even when they conflict. Awareness of values is important for the healthy running of such teams. But such teams also engage with others, and awareness of the potential for different values is always crucial.

Introduction

In the last chapter, we established the importance of relationships generally: we inevitably stand in relationship with others, and this becomes even more important in connection with people with dementia. This is no less important when it comes to questions of working together. In this chapter, we make the same broadening move: we have to see the person with dementia as situated in a variety of contexts. One such context is that of the team with whom the person is involved. But teams are not entirely circumscribed (which needs to be explained), and just as the person with dementia is situated in a variety of contexts, so, too, are there likely to be various teams involved in thinking about how to enable the person to live well. All of these teams must work together, but as we have already described, the individuals within the teams and the teams themselves will have a range of values. Navigating and negotiating values within teams and between teams is a crucial part of the process of values-based practice (VBP). For instance, there are important values around the vexed notion of confidentiality in dementia care, which we shall explore. As dementia progresses, so can the complexity of care that is required. This process can easily mean that the person with dementia is lost (a further statement which needs to be explained). This chapter will explore working together, with a view to the possibility of diverse and conflicting values. Our argument will be that we should start and finish with the person with dementia, but not forget family carers as well. The challenge for all concerned is to work together to realize the person's values and rights, despite any barriers to achieving this in practice. We shall start with a case scenario.

Vignette – Betty Price (1)

Betty Price and the Worry about Abuse

When Betty Price was referred to the old age mental health team, it was because of her behaviour, which was increasingly challenging for the staff at Homewood Residential Care Home. She had been in Homewood for just over a year and had seemed settled. But during the course of several months she had become increasingly more agitated and aggressive. The general practitioner (GP) had checked her for a chest infection, and a urine sample was negative for infection. Betty still remained disturbed and was hitting out at staff, especially during personal interventions, when she would also scream. The GP prescribed her a low dose of a drug called trazodone, which she knew had been used before in this sort of circumstance with good effect. It did not help, and Betty was more unsteady and slightly sleepy, so the GP referred her to the local old age psychiatry team.

When she was seen, she told Dr Pincus, a female psychiatrist, that men were abusing her in the shower, dragging her there to do 'terrible things'. She said she wanted to get out of the place and get back to her own home. It was clear that Betty had advanced dementia: she was disoriented and showed evidence of marked problems coordinating her movements in response to commands. This looked like dyspraxia, and she also had dysphasic (or language) problems. She remained agitated and anxious much of the time.

What Next?

Dr Pincus knew she must raise the issue of the alleged abuse with the manager of the care home. The manager, Dave Thornton, asserted that no men were involved in the personal care of Betty Price. As she was being shown out of the home, however, a care worker, who had accompanied Dr Pincus when she saw Betty, said that on night shift there was a male carer who was sometimes on duty on Betty's floor. Dr Pincus left Homewood but pondered matters as she drove back to her hospital base.

There were two problems to be considered: first, the alleged abuse; second, the behaviour which was still proving very challenging.

Dr Pincus arrived at the hospital by chance at the same time as her good social work colleague, John Bobienski. On discussing the case whilst still in the car park, they immediately agreed that even though it could easily be that Betty either was misinterpreting events or was perhaps dreaming or hallucinating, a safeguarding alert should be put in to the local council for the matter to be considered more broadly. They also felt that it would be better for Dave the manager to be given the opportunity to do this, because this would also allow some clarification as to whether or not a male carer worked on Betty's floor. Dr Pincus spoke with Dave, and he agreed that he would look into matters and, whatever the outcome as far as the male carer was concerned, he would put the safeguarding alert in regardless to cover himself and the home. He also agreed that it would be prudent for him and his staff – John had suggested that Dr Pincus should mention this – to re-write Betty's care plans around personal care to state specifically that male carers should never be involved and that there should be two carers at all times in case accusations were made.

Taking Stock

In one sense, what has happened so far is not very remarkable. It is routine as far as good practice goes. But a closer look should notice the complexity which underlies this sort of routine practice. Two doctors have now been involved: one (the GP) has played an important role in excluding physical conditions which might have accounted for the change in Betty's behaviour and has then made a decision to refer her to the psychiatrist; the psychiatrist has confirmed the diagnosis of advanced dementia and has elicited a complaint, which might reflect either psychopathology or possible abuse. The psychiatrist has then appreciated the opportunity to discuss the matter with a trusted social work colleague, which in turn has led to further liaison with the care home and a referral to the safeguarding team.

We have glided over the important role of the carer in the home who, in a sense, blew the whistle by pointing out that there was a male carer occasionally working on Betty's floor, which was obviously an important piece of information.

As things stand, values do not seem to be prominent, but, of course, they are at play. The doctors and the social worker share important values around their concerns for Betty. In so doing they are also respecting her rights, which must be valued: her rights to be cared for appropriately, to be taken seriously, to be protected from potential harms, and so forth. Shared values are also seen in the respect shown towards the safeguarding process. In these circumstances, involving the safeguarding team is felt to be important. This partly reflects trust which has been built up over several years. Dr Pincus and John Bobienski are confident that the safeguarding team will only apply a light touch, if this is all that is required, and would only escalate matters if this were necessary. Dr Pincus and John are part of the same team, social workers having been embedded in the old age psychiatry service many years before, which is part of the reason they feel comfortable and confident sharing information and making joint decisions. Part of working in the same team means that there is a raft of shared values, which are mostly taken for granted but are at work in the background.

We said at the start of the chapter that we would need to explain what we meant by saying that teams are not circumscribed. What we meant will, by now, be immediately obvious. The mental health team interacts with the team at Homewood, but also now with the safeguarding team, who in turn interacts with the care home; meanwhile, we should not forget the general practice (or primary care) team. Each of these teams will have their own values, many of which will coincide, but there is the potential for both intra- and inter-team values diversity. An example of the complexity of providing care to the population of people with dementia living in care homes is set out in Figure 7.1. What is apparent is both that (a) good coordination and communication are of paramount importance and (b) the possibility of different values emerging is not far-fetched.

Confidentiality

One important value which must be shared within and between teams is that of confidentiality. Different professional bodies issue different guidance on confidentiality, but

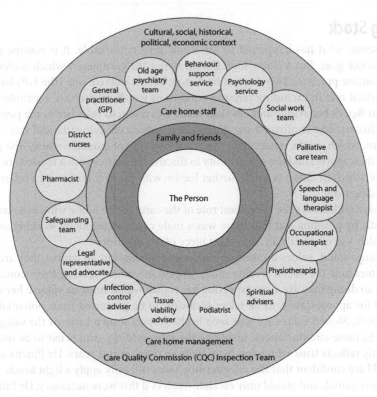

Figure 7.1 Complexity surrounding the person in the care home

luckily the guidance is very similar, showing the extent to which this is a shared value (see Box 7.1). Surprisingly, confidentiality in the context of dementia is not frequently discussed in detail. All of the guidance tends to say that if the person lacks capacity to make a decision about whether or not personal information should be shared or disclosed, then decisions should be made in the person's best interests. (The guidance in Box 7.1 in this regard largely reflects UK law, but in particular the MCA, which governs England and Wales. There are likely to be subtle differences in similar guidance in other jurisdictions.) On meeting Betty, Dr Pincus made an immediate decision that she lacked capacity to make decisions about many aspects of her care. But this was not tested in a formal manner. Betty is unaware that the information she gave to Dr Pincus has been shared with the manager of Homewood, a social worker, and the safeguarding team. We would hazard a guess that most professionals, faced by someone with advanced dementia, would take action in much the same way as Dr Pincus. This in itself shows the extent to which the relevant values are shared. It does not, however, manifest a particular concern for the rights of the person with dementia.

The UN Convention on the Rights of Persons with Disabilities, which has already been mentioned in Chapters 2 and 6, for example, would have us go further (UN, 2006). Article 12(2) states:

> States Parties shall recognize that persons with disabilities enjoy legal capacity on an equal basis with others in all aspects of life.

Box 7.1 Guidance on Confidentiality

General Medical Council (GMC) (2009)
In a section on sharing information within the health care team or with others providing care, GMC guidance states:

> Most patients understand and accept that information must be shared within the healthcare team in order to provide their care. You should make sure information is readily available to patients explaining that, unless they object, personal information about them will be shared within the healthcare team, including administrative and other staff who support the provision of their care. (paragraph 25)

The guidance goes on to say:

> You must make sure that anyone you disclose personal information to understands that you are giving it to them in confidence, which they must respect. All staff members receiving personal information in order to provide or support care are bound by a legal duty of confidence, whether or not they have contractual or professional obligations to protect confidentiality. (paragraph 28)

In connection with people who lack capacity to consent to disclosure, the guidance states:

> If you believe that a patient may be a victim of neglect or physical, sexual or emotional abuse, and that they lack capacity to consent to disclosure, you must give information promptly to an appropriate responsible person or authority, if you believe that the disclosure is in the patient's best interests or necessary to protect others from a risk of serious harm. If, for any reason, you believe that disclosure of information is not in the best interests of a neglected or abused patient, you should discuss the issues with an experienced colleague. If you decide not to disclose information, you should document in the patient's record your discussions and the reasons for deciding not to disclose. You should be prepared to justify your decision. (paragraph 63)

Nursing and Midwifery Council (NMC) (2015)
In their Code which covers professional standards of practice, the NMC states that the nurse should:

> Share necessary information with other healthcare professionals and agencies only when the interests of patient safety and public protection override the need for confidentiality. (paragraph 5.4)

Health and Care Professions Council (HCPC) (2008)
The HCPC covers a broad range of professionals, from occupational therapists to speech and language therapists, social workers in England, and so on (social workers in the other parts of the UK have different regulatory bodies). Their guidance is quite straightforward:

> Your duty to respect and protect the confidentiality of service users at all times is both a professional and a legal responsibility. (p. 7)

They also give a full account of duties around sharing within teams: 'One of the most common reasons for disclosing confidential information will be when you liaise with other health and care practitioners. This might include discussing a case with a colleague or referring a service user to another health and care practitioner. Sharing information is often part of good practice. Care is rarely provided by just one health and care practitioner, and sharing information within the multidisciplinary team is often an important way of making sure care can be provided effectively. Most service users will understand the importance of sharing information with members of the multidisciplinary team, so you will normally have implied consent to do this. However, when you share information with other colleagues, you should make sure that:

• It is necessary to provide the information and the information you provide is relevant;

- The professional receiving the information understands why you are sharing it and that they have a duty to keep it confidential; and
- You explain to the service user the possible effect of not sharing information about their care or other services you are providing. (pp. 10–11)'

They recognize, however, that it will not always be possible to gain consent for disclosure:

> In circumstances where it is not possible to get consent ... you may have to disclose information if it is in the best interests of the service user. (p. 13)

Health and Social Care Information Centre (HSCIC) (2013)

More recently, in a guide published by the HSCIC, rules around confidentiality are set out. Rule 2 is as follows:

> Members of a care team should share confidential information when it is needed for the safe and effective care of an individual.

In connection with safeguarding, they say:

> The need to share confidential information becomes an absolute imperative in cases involving a threat to the safety of others. An example of this could be the prevention of abuse of a vulnerable elderly person. This may necessitate the sharing of confidential information with the police or other organisations. (p. 15)

An Afterword

Confidentiality regarding adult safeguarding issues is now governed in many countries by the law, e.g. in England by the Care Act 2014, but with similar legislation in Wales and Scotland; see: www.scie.org.uk/care-act-2014/safeguarding-adults/

The challenge here is that there is a tendency for the diagnosis of dementia to overshadow concern about the person's rights. It might simply be accepted that Betty Price and others like her with advanced dementia would not have the requisite decision-making capacity, even with support, to consent to their confidential information being disclosed to others. The trouble with this is that it goes against basic principles enshrined in the MCA, namely that capacity should be presumed, that people should be helped to make decisions with capacity if this is possible, and that no one should be deemed to lack capacity on the grounds of a diagnosis or age, or on the basis of any other status, but only on the grounds that they fail a specific test of capacity.

One of the benefits of the multidisciplinary team (MDT) is that the appropriateness of any decisions or actions being taken are open to challenge by members of the team. This is predicated on the team running in a healthy manner and not being dominated by one individual or profession. Multi-team working can also lend support to the consensual view that information should be shared. If Dave, the manager of Homewood, had considered that Dr Pincus was being too heavy-handed in her approach, he could have objected or made a complaint. John Bobienski, the social worker, could have advised Dr Pincus not to take matters further if he considered it was inappropriate for her to do so. Finally, the safeguarding team could have refused the referral and even raised a concern about Dr Pincus's judgement if they felt she was acting in an egregious manner. But none of this happened because the values around Betty's care were shared.

In a more marginal case – someone with advanced dementia yet not as cognitively impaired as Betty – the person might specifically say that no fuss should be made. Professionals might still have a duty nonetheless, according to their codes of practice or

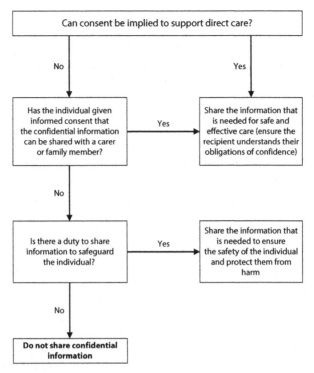

Figure 7.2 Deciding whether to share confidential information for direct care
From: Health and Social Care Information Centre (2013), p. 15 (Figure 1)

practice guidelines (see Box 7.1), to involve others if they felt that the issue represented a risk to public safety. Someone might say they do not want a fuss made about a minor incident, but if it were caused by a suspected abuser, the worry about broader public safety means action must be taken.

The concern with rights, however, should not be dismissed too lightly. The guidance from the Health and Social Care Information Centre (2013) sets out a useful algorithm for deciding when confidential information should and should not be shared, which appears in modified form in Figure 7.2.

From this it can be seen that in the case of someone like Betty, where there is a suspicion of abuse, the onus is on sharing information. If, however, someone has the capacity to give informed consent and does not do so and where there is no duty to share information for safeguarding purposes, confidential information should not be shared. But we should note that this involves three questions which raise the possibility of value judgements: Does the person lack capacity? Is she able to give informed consent (she may have capacity but be under some form of coercion; for example, she may think she is at risk of further abuse)? Is there a duty to share information (for example, in a case where there was some doubt)? We can imagine in response to the last question there being disagreement in the MDT, with one person thinking that the incident in question was too minor or uncertain to warrant referral to the safeguarding team and someone else thinking that it is always better in these circumstances to err on the side of caution. It is not always apparent that assessments of capacity involve evaluative judgements, but they do: think, for instance, of the value judgements involved in deciding whether or not the person has recalled the relevant information (how do we decide exactly what or how much information is relevant to a particular decision?) or whether or not he or she has weighed it up appropriately (Greener et al., 2012). So to follow the algorithm of Figure 7.2 will require, albeit facts will be relevant, a number of possible value judgements. And this in turn allows the possibility of disputed values, especially where there is values diversity.

Before moving away from the topic of confidentiality, it is worth noting the tensions around it, particularly early on in dementia, when the person affected might wish to retain control, including control of personal information. Generally, the rights of the person with dementia must be upheld, even if a moment might come when the rights of others to be informed start to intervene. This is how the Nuffield Council on Bioethics (2009) make this point:

> Whilst the principle of patient confidentiality is an important one in the doctor-patient relationship, a diagnosis of dementia has important implications not only for the person with dementia, but also for close family members who are likely to take on a significant caring role and need appropriate information and support to do so. (paragraph 12, pp. xix–xx)

The Nuffield Council's approach, therefore, is to recommend that a careful assessment be made of the person's ability to consent to their information being shared. If they lacked this capacity, then it might be (but it might not be) in their best interests for some information to be shared. On the whole, if they have the capacity to decide, then their information should dealt with in accordance with their wishes. In some circumstances, however, even where the person has the required capacity, the seriousness of the information (e.g. if a life were at risk or the person was subject to some form of abuse as defined by law) might mean that safeguarding measures need to be pursued with or without the person's permission. Here we see societal values trumping personal values. Informed teams, working openly, allow the tensions between such values to be brought out and weighed. Confidentiality, therefore, is an important issue involving values which may need to be negotiated in particular cases.

Vignette - Betty Price (2): Continuing Care

The safeguarding team investigated matters in the case of Betty Price. It transpired that there was a male carer in Homewood who had worked on Betty's floor on two specific nights because of a lack of staff. During the day there are also male care workers on the floor, but there are enough female carers that a male carer would never be required to be involved in intimate care of a female resident. There is no record to suggest that on the nights in question Betty required intimate care from the male care worker. He is, in any case, well known in the home, with a good reputation and unblemished record. The safeguarding team were happy enough not to pursue matters, but to leave Dr Pincus to follow up with Mrs Price and report again if anything further were to occur that was of concern.

Dr Pincus did indeed see Betty Price again. On this occasion, there was no mention of possible abuse, but instead Betty described people talking to her through the pipes in the ceiling, telling her that people were trying to kill her. This sounded more like a psychosis to Dr Pincus. It seemed as if, in response to psychotic phenomena (that is, experiences of which others were not aware), Betty was remaining agitated and aggressive. Dr Pincus asked her colleagues from the Behaviour Support Service to see Betty more regularly and to carry out an assessment in order to try to formulate a behavioural plan to help with management of the agitation and aggression. Minu Ganesh was the CPN from the Behaviour Support Service who took on the task.

Having liaised closely with Betty's two daughters and with Kim Magday, who is the senior care worker on the floor in Homewood where Betty is a resident, Minu came up with a detailed support plan, which was developed as part of a formulation session involving all concerned in Betty's care. It suggested that activities which might be meaningful to Betty (such as looking at pictures of country houses, which her daughter said she always enjoyed doing) should be used to engage her in the hope that this would distract her and add to her sense of well-being. It was also said that she enjoyed listening to Barry Manilow recordings. Staff were asked to spend at least ten minutes giving Betty one-to-one attention both in the morning and the evening: just being with her to talk or stroke her hand. Plans were also made to help keep Betty oriented to the time and the day and month of the year, as well as to where she was and who the people around her were. Staff were to make sure that they introduced themselves and to inform Betty before undertaking any tasks with her. A detailed care plan around personal intervention was also reviewed and updated and all the staff were familiarized with the plan. This included the suggestion that staff should try to engage Betty in day-to-day (non-challenging) conversation before introducing the idea that they were going to provide intimate or personal care. Kim also arranged for a further mid-stream urine (MSU) to be collected, to exclude infection, and both pain charts and bowel charts were to be used to make sure that neither pain nor constipation were causing her distress.

Why the Detail?

It would be reasonable to wonder why we have given so much detail about the content of Betty's behaviour support plan. There are four reasons:

- As we discussed in the previous chapter, a central tenet of values-based practice is that it should be person-centred. This means that Betty Price must be central to our concerns, but also that we should know about her in detail, taking a broad view of what might count for Betty, partly in order to know what she would have valued.
- This broad view means that we must think about her physical state as well as about her psychological, social, and spiritual needs (and so on). An infection, constipation or pain might all contribute to disturbances in her mental state. In part, this helps to remind us of the connections between VBP and evidence-based practice (EBP). As originally defined, evidence-based medicine (EBM) was conceived as involving the integration of the best research evidence, clinical expertise, *and patient values* (Sackett et al., 2000). We know from research and from clinical experience that infections, pain, and constipation (amongst other things) are potent causes of agitation in people with advanced dementia, partly because they might cause delirium as an added complication. Hence, good practice guides highlight the assessment and treatment of medical conditions, the appropriate use of analgesia, and the efficacy of non-pharmacological interventions (Alzheimer's Society, 2013).
- In emphasizing the breadth of the behaviour support plan, we are also advertising an approach to the management of behaviour that people find challenging (James and Jackman, 2017). This approach is itself predicated, in

part, on aspects of person-centred practice, which (as we have seen) is a vital component of VBP. It involves getting to know as fully as possible the story or narrative of the person concerned in order to understand in what way (or ways) his or her needs are not being met. Of course, a person's narrative is everything about them, involving personality before and after the onset of the condition, their beliefs, wishes, feelings and values, and so on. This, in turn, is predicated on the view that when people with dementia present behaviour that others find challenging, it is highly likely that this reflects unmet needs. The task is then to identify the needs, which will only be done by knowing the individual well (Hughes and Beatty, 2013).

- The notion of knowing the person's narrative stresses the ways in which we, too, as professionals become involved as actors in the narrative, with all that this entails. This chimes with the theme of this chapter. For what we see is the way in which, to provide Betty with appropriate care, different teams must work together to provide coherence to the ongoing story. The Behaviour Support Service (represented by Minu Ganesh) works with the team from Homewood (represented by Kim Magday). Moreover, the teams must include others, not just Dr Pincus and the GP, but also Betty's daughters. The emphasis is on working together to share knowledge to improve the situation for Betty. As in the definition of EBM alluded to earlier, this must involve Betty's values insofar as we can ascertain what these might have been and what they would be now. Up to this point things have gone smoothly because the values of all concerned, including the teams, have been shared.

This is not quite true actually, because initially Minu found that the Homewood team were not familiar with the model she was using. They did not recognize that Betty might have unmet needs; instead, some of them saw much of her behaviour as wilful. Some education of the staff was required alongside the development of the behaviour support plan. The behaviour of staff, other residents, the physical environment, the care home regimen, and other factors may all play a part in inadvertently causing or exacerbating behaviour that challenges or distresses (Kitwood, 1997). Part of the aim of the education was to bring the values of the teams into alignment. The teams needed to understand that Betty would not hitherto have behaved in these ways, so there is something going on for Betty which needs attention.

A final point to note, however, is the important underpinning role played in all of this by rights. Behaviour that challenges is, according to the approach we are commending, usually a reflection of unmet needs. But needs are often based on rights. My need to be allowed out to walk is a reflection of a variety of underpinning rights: my right to self-determination, to liberty, to a private life, and so on. We could say, then, that behaviour that challenges should frequently alert us to the possibility of rights being abused in some way. One of the benefits of multidisciplinary teams is that they may be more likely to be sensitive to not just the variety of values in play but also the importance of the rights that are at risk in some circumstances.

Vignette - Betty Price (3): To Use or Not to Use?

Minu and Kim worked closely to implement the behaviour support plan. Things improved to a degree, and certainly the staff at Homewood felt less stressed by the situation, but

Betty was still agitated most days and could still be violent at times, both verbally and, during personal interventions, physically. She was already receiving a variety of medicines for her physical and mental state, including an antidepressant and a sleeping tablet. The staff were also using lorazepam, an anxiolytic drug, to calm her when she was agitated. This helped but left her drowsy and at risk of falling. Minu started to feel that the risk of falling was too great, because the staff were inclined to use the lorazepam too frequently. But if the lorazepam were to be stopped, the staff would feel less secure. Meanwhile, Betty was still shouting when agitated, apparently in response to auditory hallucinations, and she seemed suspicious almost all the time. She talked openly about delusions which seemed to be associated with the hallucinations: about people coming to get her and about dead bodies being moved at night. Minu started to feel that it might be worthwhile trying some medication for this and, in the past, they had had some success in using the antidementia drug memantine.

Dr Pincus was not too keen to prescribe memantine. She agreed with Minu that it had seemed helpful in the past, but she was aware that the evidence base to support its use for agitation was not strong. In any case, it seemed to her that the more likely diagnosis for Mrs Price was that of vascular dementia, for which memantine is not licensed. Dr Pincus was aware of the evidence that antipsychotics have 'modest but significant benefits in the treatment of aggression and psychosis', at least in Alzheimer's disease (Ballard, Corbett, and Howard, 2014); and the treatment with an antipsychotic seemed justified on the grounds that Betty's needs involved the relief of these disturbing experiences and thoughts, which the behavioural plan on its own had not settled. Nevertheless, antipsychotics can increase morbidity and mortality in people with dementia. Some of the other members of the community MDT also raised concerns that the antipsychotic would make it more likely that Betty would fall and be sedated. They also felt that it would divert the care home staff from the behavioural approach, making it easy for them to rely on the medication rather than to give time to Betty in a more person-centred manner. Dr Pincus felt, however, that this was a case where the risks of the antipsychotic were outweighed by the possible benefits and, in any case, she would use the lowest possible efficacious dose in a drug with the best side effect profile and review its use after a few months (Ballard et al., 2014). This was partly on the grounds that Dr Pincus had been sure all along that Betty was experiencing true hallucinations, rather than just misperceptions, so the antipsychotic seemed to be indicated – it was not simply being used as a matter of trial and error.

The decision to use the antipsychotic followed a discussion in the multidisciplinary meeting, which helped to clarify the competing facts but also set out people's different values. Some of these values were conflicting: on the one hand, antipsychotics were still valued as drugs which could be used to good effect in dementia; on the other hand, the possible side effects of the drugs, with the risk even of death, meant that the drugs were generally given less value in dementia. But best practice approaches had already been tried and had not yet been sufficient, and Betty was still seeming to suffer from her hallucinations and associated delusional beliefs. She seemed to be the sort of person who might benefit from the antipsychotic, which could be used according to good practice guidelines (Alzheimer's Society, 2013). The family agreed, with the risks having been discussed with them, that the antipsychotic was worth trying, and Minu was determined to continue to work with Kim to see that the behavioural support plan was being followed.

All in all, there was a consensus that this was the next step, albeit the whole team was aware of the concerns about the risks which had been openly aired in discussion.

An important part of values-based practice within the MDT is that there should be mutual respect: the concerns about the use of the antipsychotic were certainly out on the table during the team meeting and were understood. None was disvalued. And inasmuch as the concerns (reflecting the different values associated with the different risks) were still in play, this would be an example of dissensus in values-based practice (Fulford et al., 2012; see especially Chapter 13). It was not that one view had come to dominate and had been accepted wholeheartedly by all. Indeed, no one in the team thought there was a single clear answer to the problem. But they were all happy that a right process had been followed and that nothing had been overlooked. It was a *democratic* process in the sense that everyone's concerns had been heard, and it was a *transparent* process, the results of which had been shared beyond the team (e.g. with the family and with the staff at Homewood). The reasons for the decision were clear, as were the doubts.

Different Team Values

We are certainly not advocating the general use of antipsychotics for agitation and aggression in dementia. Behavioural approaches are the preferred option. But in particular circumstances, drug therapies of various sorts might be useful. Nor are we suggesting that differences in values can always be accommodated so easily within or between teams. As it happened, in the case of Betty Price, no one was very upset by the decision to try an antipsychotic, given the particular circumstances. There can be, however, quite marked differences in outlook.

This is shown, for instance, in an interesting study of the different ethical views seen in Kerala in southern India compared to The Netherlands (Sowmini and de Vries, 2009).

Before considering this study (which shows differences) in a little more detail, however, it is worth pausing to notice the similarities between the use of MDTs in both India and Europe. It is commonplace in, say, the UK, as it is in India, to find that MDTs will have a unified purpose. Shaji (2010) describes using an MDT in the Urban Community Dementia Care Services (UCDS) project, between 1996 and 1999, which aimed to identify people with dementia, provide services, train community health workers, organize support, and encourage research. There was a strong commitment to the values of the project. The importance of the MDT in terms of improving specialist services in Kerala continues to be recognized (Kumar et al., 2015). In addition, what we see, both in the examples from a high-income country such as the UK (in which people like Betty Price live) and in projects in low- and middle-income countries (Shaji, 2010), is the importance of the MDT reaching out to involve others in the community. The strategy in Kerala must be to develop 'a pool of community workers and dementia friends to provide care and support at the point of need' (Kumar et al., 2015). Thus, we see the MDT of values-based practice being, to use Fulford et al.'s terminology, both 'extended in form (extending to non-clinical as well as clinical team members) as well as function (extending to team values as well as team knowledge and skills)' (Fulford et al., 2012: 127).

To return to the comparative study, both Kerala and The Netherlands have ageing populations and an increasing prevalence of dementia. But their cultures are very different. The researchers found quite marked differences between Kerala and The Netherlands in terms of advance care planning and end-of-life decision making (Sowmini and de

Vries, 2009). The study emphasizes the ways in which cultural values affect attitudes and approaches towards the ethical issues that emerge in the context of dementia. The authors suggested ways in which the two cultures might learn from each other. For instance, in Kerala dementia is more likely to be seen as part of natural ageing, whereas in The Netherlands it is seen as an organic brain disease. It might help the Indian population to regard dementia as a disease like other diseases, but it might help the Europeans not to over-medicalize dementia and instead to take a more holistic view. Over-medicalization is, perhaps, part of the reason it can be difficult to get care homes to pursue a psychosocial approach to behavioural problems in dementia with any vigour, because there is an underlying belief that tablets are a better solution. Medicine is, in this sense, valued more highly. In The Netherlands, institutional care was more common, whereas in Kerala, home-based care was the norm. The authors recommended '[a] balancing of the institutional and the familial, the formal and the relational' with greater attention to 'the deeper personal and emotional dimensions' of the person (Sowmini and de Vries, 2009). On the one hand, the use of advance directives was clearly valued in The Netherlands; on the other, 'relational embeddedness' in Kerala promotes 'an atmosphere of care that is gratifying and comprehensive'. The Dutch model of end-of-life care encourages a non-aggressive approach over a more paternalistic model of medical practice in Kerala. But in Kerala the issue of euthanasia 'remains totally alien', whereas the Dutch system has embraced it, which is ascribed to differences in cultural and religious worldviews (Sowmini and de Vries, 2009).

So we can see quite different values at play between different teams reflecting different cultures. But even in a country such as the UK, which is multi-cultural, MDTs might well have markedly different values when it comes to issues that arise at the end of life.

Vignette - Betty Price (4): To Admit or Not to Admit?

Betty Price did very well on the antipsychotic in that her behaviour settled: she was hardly ever agitated and the aggression disappeared. She was able to smile and react appropriately to the carers. Kim Magday and the other staff at Homewood found her much easier to engage with and all seemed well. It was after only a few months, however, that she started to seem increasingly frail. She took to her bed and it was very difficult to get her up at all: she had to be hoisted and she seemed unable to walk. Betty was much less interested in food and drink, so this was also a daily concern for staff and family.

The dose of the antipsychotic was reduced and then it was stopped. Luckily the previous behaviour did not return; but nor did Betty improve. The GP and Dr Pincus wondered whether she had had a small stroke: her face seemed a little drooped on one side, towards which she was also leaning. (Perhaps, after all, this was caused by the antipsychotic.) Her daughters said they thought she should be in hospital; some of the staff agreed, but some said that this was her home and she was better off being cared for in her home. These staff thought that nothing different would be done in a hospital that they could not do for her. The GP was not very keen to have her admitted to hospital. The psychiatry team felt that some clarity over the diagnosis might be helpful to all concerned, but also felt that the hospital would be a confusing environment for her and was likely to make her more agitated again. They recommended involving the community palliative care team, who agreed that it sounded as if there might have been a vascular event, in other words, a small stroke. They were also worried about Betty's swallowing, because she was now coughing when she had a drink (which was not often). The speech and language therapist agreed to come to see Betty and felt that her swallowing was compromised to a degree. They raised a question about some form of tube feeding, both because of her dysphagia (swallowing difficulties) and to maintain her body weight to make pressure sores less likely. Betty's daughters now felt even more strongly that an admission to hospital was necessary.

It was decided that, since she lacked the capacity to make decisions concerning either a hospital admission or artificial feeding, decisions should be made in her best interests. A meeting was arranged at Homewood for all those involved. In the first part of the meeting, once the current clinical facts were set out, it was agreed that everyone should say exactly what they thought. This revealed a number of understandable concerns and, incidentally, a diversity of values: from those who felt that everything that could be done should be done, to those who felt that any intervention was likely to be burdensome for Betty. The one shared value was that everyone wanted to do the best they could for Betty – it was just that there were different ideas about what 'the best' might mean. At any rate, it was clear that Betty was to be the centre of concern. At the start of the chapter we suggested that complexity can sometimes lead to the person getting lost. This can happen if people are more concerned to be defensive, or to defend their patches (turf wars), or to protect their budgets, or to pass the buck and make sure that problems fall on the shoulders of someone else. These sorts of concerns are typically a reflection of other values, where the people concerned believe the values that lie behind their concerns are the 'right' ones. Everyone accepted there was considerable uncertainty, but in the course of the discussion three key things emerged, two about evidence and one about an ethical approach:

1. There was evidence that admission to hospital in people with advanced dementia did not do much good: investigations were likely to be undertaken which would not change the course of events and, indeed, some evidence to suggest that mortality was quite high amongst people with advanced dementia admitted in this way (Sampson et al., 2009a).
2. There was not much evidence that tube feeding did any good in people with advanced dementia. Indeed, most of the things a tube might be thought to prevent, such as weight loss or aspiration (i.e. secretions or food going into the lungs), still occurred in dementia (Sampson et al., 2009b).
3. In ethical terms, it can be argued that where there is little evidence that an investigation or intervention would be efficacious and where it is likely that it would be burdensome to the person, there is no moral obligation to pursue the procedure (which might include hospital admission).

Betty's daughters were placated by these thoughts. But they were still worried, as were the staff from Homewood, that Betty's care needs might not be met unless she went into hospital. The district nurse and the Macmillan nurse from the palliative care team were able to reassure them that they would be providing support, both monitoring her physical needs and supporting the residential care home staff if any more complicated interventions were required. For instance, the district nurse said that they could provide some help if Betty were to require subcutaneous fluid to augment her oral fluid intake; she could also ask the GP to prescribe some supplements to help to maintain Betty's weight. The Macmillan nurse said that there were no immediate palliative care needs, but she would be able to facilitate the drawing up of a 'Treatment Escalation Plan', to set out when an admission would be necessary, for example, if there were to be a nasty fracture or something else untoward which would benefit from attention in the hospital. She also said that she would liaise with the speech and language therapist (who was unable to attend the meeting) to say that the staff would like more education on how to feed someone at risk of choking, as well as advice on thickened fluids for Betty to help prevent her from aspirating. By the end of the meeting there remained uncertainty and some worries, but Betty's daughters and the staff at Homewood were more confident that the right things were being done, and would be done, and that they would be able to express their opinions as circumstances changed.

Working Together

There is no guarantee that having an MDT will bring about good outcomes. There is at least the possibility, however, that different voices will (if they are heard) lead to more considered outcomes. When an MDT works on values-based practice principles, however, the likelihood of a good outcome is increased. But by this we must understand that a 'good' outcome does not mean that all will go well. Nor, as we have seen, does it mean that a consensus precludes the possibility of different opinions still being held, even if there has been agreement on the way forward. Dissenting opinions, reflecting diverse and conflicting values, can still be acknowledged openly. At least in values-based practice these differences and concerns can be openly faced and discussed, rather than fester unacknowledged. So values-based practice allows us to work together honestly, with candour.

Moreover, we have seen that the values that count are neither confined to the individual, nor to the MDT, but extend beyond the team, to other teams and to those involved who are not in teams, to clients or carers trying to make sense of what is happening. The commitment to respect values within a team inevitably suggests a commitment to respect the values of anyone conscientiously involved in a person's care, so that a process of good communication follows with a commitment to make the person affected central. Values-based practice encourages working together in an inclusive manner.

The insistence on the importance of values, as we have seen in the earlier debate about the antipsychotic and again in the debate about whether or not Betty should be admitted to hospital, does not preclude the equal importance of facts: if there is evidence, it, too, must be on the table if the (extended) team is to function well and if the values are to be applied prudently. Values-based practice makes us work together with a broad, full-field perspective of facts as well as values (Fulford, 1989).

To return to the principles of our Manifesto:

- Dementia is a unique touchstone for understanding the human condition: we are interconnected and interdependent, so we must work together in a spirit of openness and mutual regard;
- Dementia as disease emphasizes the facts that surround our physical being (from constipation to abnormal neurochemistry), and dementia as disability emphasizes the rights, which we all share, that safeguard people living with dementia;
- VBP and an awareness of rights provide an essential framework for providing support, care, and treatment to people with dementia, their families, and their friends: MDTs must be aware of how values (shared and disputed) as well as rights shape the care that they must give.

Conclusion

We have seen that in MDTs values are at play even when actions and decisions seem uncontroversial. Shared values permeate practice. Both individuals and teams have values, which may be shared or diverse. MDTs need to be very aware of the need for confidential information to be respected. The need to share information should not be blind to the need to uphold the person's right to confidentiality. Processes and procedures must be followed by MDTs, as they must by individuals, in order to show proper respect for the rights of those who cannot defend their own rights.

Taking a broad view of the person not only means being aware of his or her values but also means proper attention should be paid to the biological facts relevant to the case. More broadly, values-based practice does not preclude evidence-based practice and, indeed, demands it. Understanding the person broadly (knowing the narrative), in any case, forms a basic tenet of good management of behaviour that is challenging in dementia, but this is underpinned by a respect for the person's rights.

Of course, working in an MDT will not always involve consensus, but it is better for dissensus to be open, that is, for contrasting values to be acknowledged and for the right approach to be taken in dealing with dissent in a transparent manner. Different teams will reflect different cultures, so there is the possibility of dissensus between teams, but nonetheless, the same respect should be shown between teams as within them. Extended teams will include non-clinicians as well as clinicians, and teams will also act as a repository of knowledge and skill, and of values.

Teams must work together, but the person with dementia must remain the focus of all that teams do and decide, albeit recognizing that the person is located in a nexus of relationships that must be taken seriously and included in an appropriate fashion in the work of the team.

Key Points

- Values, shared and diverse, permeate the work of individuals and of teams.
- Confidentiality should be a key value of MDTs, albeit information must be shared, since it reflects a person's basic rights.
- We can respect rights by following proper processes and procedures.
- Values-based practice does not preclude evidence-based practice and, indeed, demands it: teams should be repositories of knowledge and skill, as well as of values.
- Different teams reflect different cultures, so there is the possibility of *dissensus* between teams.
- Dissenting views and values need to be acknowledged, heard, and discussed in an open manner if teams are to operate efficiently, effectively, and reflect basic human rights.
- Teams should not be essentially closed, but open to include non-clinicians as well as clinicians.
- The person with dementia – with his or her nexus of relationships – must remain the focus of all that teams do.

References

Alzheimer's Society. (2013). *Optimising Treatment and Care for Behavioural and Psychological Symptoms of Dementia*. London: Alzheimer's Society.

Ballard, C., Corbett, A., and Howard, R. (2014). Prescription of antipsychotics in people with dementia. *British Journal of Psychiatry* **205**: 4–5. doi: 10.1192/bjp .bp.113.128710

Fulford, K. W. M. (1989). *Moral Theory and Medical Practice*. Cambridge: Cambridge University Press.

Fulford, K. W. M. (Bill), Peile, E., and Carroll, H. (2012). *Essential Values-Based Practice: Clinical Stories Linking Science with People*. Cambridge: Cambridge University Press.

General Medical Council. (2009). *Confidentiality*. London: GMS. Available via www.gmc-uk.org/guidance (last accessed 28 December 2017).

Greener, H., Poole, M., Emmett, C., Bond, J., Louw, S. J., and Hughes, J. C. (2012). Value judgements and conceptual tensions: decision-making in relation to hospital discharge for people with dementia. *Clinical Ethics* 7, 166–74.

Health and Care Professions Council. (2008). *Confidentiality – Guidance for Registrants*. London: HCPC. Available via: www .hcpc-uk.co.uk/publications/ (last accessed 28 December 2017).

Health and Social Care Information Centre (2013). *A Guide to Confidentiality in Health and Social Care*. London: HSCIC. Available via: www.hscic gov.uk/ (last accessed 28 December 2017).

Hughes, J. C., and Beatty, A. (2013). Understanding the person with dementia: A clinicophilosophical case discussion. *Advances in Psychiatric Treatment* 19, 337–43.

James, I. A., and Jackman, L. (2017). *Understanding Behaviour in Dementia that Challenges: A Guide to Assessment and Treatment*, 2nd edn. London and Philadelphia: Jessica Kingsley Publishers.

Kitwood, T. (1997). *Dementia Reconsidered: The Person Comes First*. Buckingham: Open University Press.

Kumar, S., Varghese, B., Tharayil, H. M., and Roy, J. (2015). Dementia friendly Kerala: The way forward. *Kerala Journal of Psychiatry* **28**, 94–99.

Nursing and Midwifery Council. (2015). *The Code: Professional Standards of Practice and Behaviour for Nurses and Midwives*. London: NMC. Available via: www.nmc-uk.org (last accessed 28 December 2017).

Sackett, D. L., Straus, S. E., Scott Richardson, W., Rosenberg, W., and Haynes, R. B. (2000). *Evidence-Based Medicine: How to Practice [sic] and Teach EBM*, 2nd edn. Edinburgh and London: Churchill Livingstone.

Sampson, E. L., Blanchard, M. R., Jones, L., Tookman, A., and King, M. (2009a). Dementia in the acute hospital: Prospective cohort study of prevalence and mortality. *British Journal of Psychiatry* **195**, 61–66.

Sampson, E. L., Candy, B., and Jones, L. (2009b). Enteral tube feeding for older people with advanced dementia. *Cochrane Database of Systematic Reviews 2009*, Issue 2. Art. No.: CD007209. doi:10.1002/14651858.CD007209.pub2.

Shaji, S. (2010). Dementia care in developing countries. In J. C. Hughes, M. Lloyd-Williams, and G. A. Sachs, eds, *Supportive Care for the Person with Dementia*. Oxford: Oxford University Press, pp. 89–98.

Sowmini, C. V., and De Vries, R. (2009). A cross cultural review of the ethical issues in dementia care in Kerala, India and The Netherlands. *International Journal of Geriatric Psychiatry* **24**, 329–34.

United Nations. (2006). *Convention on the Rights of Persons with Disabilities* [A/RES/61/106]. Available via: www.un.org/development/desa/disabilities/convention-on-the-rights-of-persons-with-disabilities .html (last accessed 28 December 2017).

Chapter

8

Scientifically Speaking

Topics covered in this chapter

- This chapter explores in some detail the close relationship between facts and values.
- The pervasive nature of values is seen in the issues that arise in practice in connection with the use of cholinesterase inhibitors.
- The importance of facts *and* values is also demonstrated in a discussion of prodromal dementia, focusing mainly on mild cognitive impairment (MCI).
- We can see how there are frameworks which support our activities, made up of facts and values.
- These frameworks can be considered myths, which are useful, but which can also be dislodged.

Take-away message for practice

You must think facts; think values. The evidence around issues such as the use of medication for dementia and the investigation of early (prodromal) dementia is intriguing and crucial, but it is important to recognize that the evidence supports and is supported by evaluative judgements.

Introduction

This chapter focuses on the two-feet principle of VBP. This is captured by the slogan, introduced in Chapter 1, 'think facts; think values'. Facts and values are always together. They are partners, but it's a partnership that changes depending on the circumstances. Nevertheless, it remains a real partnership in that both facts and values can (and usually should) always be considered. We shall develop this theme in connection with a variety of scientific advances relevant to dementia care. One of the things this will help to bring out is the extent to which we all have background frameworks of beliefs and values which shape our lives. One of the benefits of the VBP approach is that it acknowledges these various background frameworks. By so doing, it improves the conversations – it makes them more honest and realistic – by making the values and facts conspicuous. Conversations that ignore conspicuous facts will be ignorant; conversations that fail to factor in values will be facile.

We shall shortly discuss two scientific advances in connection with dementia where the two-feet principle sheds some light: the use of the cholinesterase inhibitors and advances in diagnostics which allow us to characterize prodromal dementia in more detail. Both of these scientific advances must be hailed as important achievements, each of which has the potential to improve the lives of people who live with dementia. But we shall first say a little more about the two-feet principle.

Think Facts; Think Values

We might put it this way: facts are always about the world, about things in the world. It is a fact that there are estimated to be about 50 million people in the world living with dementia (Alzheimer's Disease International, 2016). It seems reasonable to ask how this fact about the world involves values. Let's start this section, however, with a more difficult case:

$$2 + 2 = 4!$$

Now, this does seem simply to be a fact. Whatever my values (we might presume) if I have two chickens and so does my partner, then we have four chickens in total. But philosophers could easily raise questions about this. (They always raise questions! After all, raising questions is what Bertrand Russell [1872–1970] said philosophy was about.[1]) A question might be about how these marks (i.e. the numerals) connect to the reality of the world. Why should '2' designate what we mean by 'two'? How is this designation achieved? Could it ever change so that '2 + 2' could equal 5?

We might regard these as silly questions! In fact (with no pun intended), they are highly complicated questions which have implications – depending on how we answer them – for how we see ourselves in the world. One possible view is that words attach themselves to objects, but this is complicated when we are dealing with abstract concepts such as numbers. Another view, associated with the philosopher Ludwig Wittgenstein (1889–1951), is that we understand the meaning of words (but also symbols) when we understand their use. To understand '2', therefore, we do not have to grasp the 'thing' designated by the number; we just have to understand the role that '2' plays in our lives. On the one view, grasping the meaning of words and symbols is akin to being a good computer, linking words to objects or pictures or other abstract entities (whatever they might be); on the other view, grasping meanings is a matter of living a particular form of life in which certain things matter and certain things just are the case.

All of this need not detain us further, and obviously philosophers would have a good deal more to say about it. However, first, it is enough to support the suggestion that even '2 + 2 = 4' reflects certain sorts of values. Values are action-guiding, as we suggested in Chapters 1 and 2, and that '2 + 2 = 4' makes us behave in certain ways and not in others

---

[1] 'Thus, to sum up our discussion of the value of philosophy: Philosophy is to be studied, not for the sake of any definite answers to its questions, since no definite answers can, as a rule, be known to be true, but rather for the sake of the questions themselves; because these questions enlarge our conception of what is possible, enrich our intellectual imagination, and diminish the dogmatic assurance which closes the mind against speculation; but above all because, through the greatness of the universe which philosophy contemplates, the mind also is rendered great, and becomes capable of that union with the universe which constitutes its highest good' (Russell, 1967: 93–94).

is enough to show that there are values associated with these facts. There is no problem, usually, around '2 + 2 = 4' because the values that underpin the relevant facts are shared. We all agree that '2 + 2 = 4' and, moreover, it is of value to us that '2' avocados means just that, so if we need four avocados, we buy two more. Second, these considerations are not totally divorced from how we think about dementia (see Hughes et al., 2006: 21–23). But that really is for another day (and see Hughes, 2011 for a fuller account of these thoughts)!

What, then, about the fact that an estimated 50 million people in the world are living with dementia? The values at play here are much more obvious. Chiefly, it depends on how the estimates have been made and on what we mean by 'dementia'. It might be thought that we all agree on what 'dementia' is or is not. Even if we do all agree, the different studies in different countries all over the world may have used slightly different methodologies and slightly different definitions or tests to assess what might or might not amount to dementia. A number of evaluative judgements must have been made in order to reach the estimated figure. The suggestion is not that those value judgements are erroneous, for they were made by experts in the field. It is just that the data chosen and the definitions or scales used could vary across the world, and evaluative judgements must be made. Even when a standard scale or set of criteria is used, we have to rely on the scale or criteria being applied in a standard way. The worker on the ground in Sri Lanka must judge that this person has failed or passed the particular test; the researcher in Canada must make the same judgement, which should be under similar circumstances (e.g. when the person is alert, not adversely affected by drugs, and so on) despite the enormous differences that might exist between the two settings; and the researcher in London looking at the Sri Lankan and Canadian data must judge that they are of sufficient quality to be included in the estimate of world prevalence. In short, the fact that 50 million people worldwide are living with dementia is a fact that involves evaluative judgements at different levels. One way to put all of this is to say that facts are value-laden. When we think facts, we must think values.

Cholinesterase Inhibitors

The acetylcholinesterase inhibitors were the first class of drugs to be used for symptomatic treatment of Alzheimer's disease. They appeared on the British market for use in the National Health Service (NHS) in 1997, so have now been around for over 20 years. There are three of them: donepezil, rivastigmine, and galantamine. (The fourth drug licensed for use in Alzheimer's disease, memantine, works in a different fashion and appeared a little later. We'll stick to discussing the first of the earlier drugs, donepezil, also known as Aricept. Much of what we say can also be said of the other drugs, but we'll use donepezil as our exemplar.) They all work in roughly the same way. They block the work of cholinesterase, which is an enzyme that encourages the breakdown of acetylcholine. Acetylcholine is a neurotransmitter in the brain. It is a chemical that is released from one nerve ending to activate the next nerve. It is broken down in the gap between the nerves by the enzyme acetylcholinesterase so that its constituent parts can be taken up again by the nerve and reused. A cholinesterase inhibitor is a drug that inhibits the work of the enzyme. The result is that the neurotransmitter continues to work in the gap between the nerves. In short, drugs such as donepezil keep the messenger chemicals in the brain working for longer.

We know that these drugs do some good in Alzheimer's disease. (They also work in some other dementias but are only licensed in the UK for Alzheimer's.) In a review of the evidence in 2011, the National Institute for Health and Care Excellence (NICE) found that the cholinesterase inhibitors were beneficial in terms of cognition; that is, in terms of memory, understanding, visuospatial abilities, and the like (NICE, 2011). This is all good news. There is some evidence, too, that donepezil is helpful in terms of function and in terms of the overall impression of change (as judged by a clinician assessing the person) caused by the dementia. However, not all of the evidence is of very good quality. For instance, the guidance quotes 'a representative from the manufacturer of donepezil' who informed the NICE committee that 'a single open-label study found an average of 17.5 months delay in the time to institutionalisation with donepezil treatment'. Whilst this result looks good, a single study, which has not yet been published (and so not yet subject to peer review), and was not in any case a controlled study, would not generally count as very good evidence.

Reflection point

Is it possible that the values of the pharmaceutical industry have permeated society and distorted the judgements of those who receive payment from 'big pharma'?

The strongest evidence is to do with cognitive function. But even here it is worth looking closely. Using the Mini-Mental State Examination (MMSE), a scale used all over the world, which mostly tests memory but also reading, writing, and copying, as well as orientation and concentration, etc., and is scored out of 30, using the overall pooled benefit in comparison with placebos, the drug improves cognition by 1.165 points at 12 weeks and by 1.206 points at 24 weeks. Both of these findings are statistically very significant ($p < .001$). So much for some of the facts.

Now let's think about values in connection with the perspective of one of us (JCH) working in old age psychiatry services in different UK locations: West Berkshire, Oxford, Newcastle upon Tyne, North Tyneside, and now Bath.

Reflection point

What is the value of a 1.206 increase on the MMSE anyway? And who should judge this?
    Even more fundamentally, the statistics ($p < .001$) suggest that there is less than a 1 in a 1,000 chance that the clinical improvement in terms of cognitive function occurred by chance. But is this a level of significance that we should value? (The answer is going to be, in all probability, yes! But we should still be clear that it's an evaluative judgement, albeit one where the values are mostly shared.)

The Clinician's Story

When donepezil first came on the market in 1997, many of us were delighted and excited. (Again, to reiterate, we're using donepezil as an example, but similar things could be said about the other drugs despite slight variations in terms of, for instance, side effects.) There had been a previous acetylcholinesterase inhibitor, tacrine, used in America, which had sadly failed because it caused liver damage. But here – in the form of donepezil – was a safe medication which produced benefits by directly tackling the effects of the pathology of Alzheimer's disease. This was an enormous breakthrough. And despite any more seemingly negative things that might be said later, the enormity of the breakthrough should not be forgotten.

> **Reflection point**
> We've said that the drugs are safe, but we lack the view of any consumers (at least here) who might have different values concerning safety.

Despite the excitement, induced in part by the drug representatives from the pharmaceutical companies coming around and showing us graphs of the data that indicated people on donepezil declined less quickly than people not on the drug, there was also some scepticism.

> **Reflection point**
> The drug reps, understandably, pushed their products quite hard when the drugs were new, so doctors had to try to maintain their values and not be overwhelmed by the values contained in the marketing material.

What difference, we asked, would a 1-point (well, to be exact, a 1.206-point) improvement on the MMSE make to someone's everyday life (actually, the original studies used another test of cognitive function)? It's the difference between knowing that it's a Tuesday in spring and the current year (but not knowing the month or exact date) and knowing that the month is actually May (but still not knowing the exact date). Perhaps on the first occasion I missed the month by a single month and said it was April when, in fact, it was May. If I have the same score on both occasions on all the other tests of the MMSE, what difference does the 1 point make? So, we had these sorts of cynical thoughts about the breakthrough represented by donepezil.

> **Reflection point**
> What were the values of patients, who may or may not think it of value always to be able to recall the exact month? Perhaps knowing the season is enough.

But, of course, some people improved by more than 1 point. Occasionally there were reports in the popular press that these medications had effected a miracle cure. We also witnessed this, but in people with dementia with Lewy bodies (DLB), where the drugs seem to work better than they do in Alzheimer's disease (but the drug companies haven't felt moved to acquire licenses for the use of the drug in DLB). In one case, the person was about to be admitted to a nursing home but improved so greatly it was possible for her to go home, where she was filmed serving tea to the television crew who came to see her.

So the drugs can work very well. But normally it isn't like this. Normally, the patient was assessed in her home before the medication and scored 17/30 on the MMSE, signifying a moderate dementia. Seen three or four months later, after treatment, she now scored 18/30. We could say, therefore, that the drug was working, because we might have expected the score to go down a little in that time. But occasionally the score was still 17/30, in which case, we could still say that the score might have gone down, so the fact that it remained constant was equivalent to the score going up. Or, perhaps, the score had gone down to 16/30, in which case, we could argue that it might have been a little lower had it not been for the donepezil, so the medication should continue. We were especially likely to make this argument if her daughter told us that the patient seemed to be coping better. Then we were more likely to say that, despite a slight fall in the MMSE, the overall clinical impression was one of improvement and hence the donepezil had proven efficacious.

Reflection point

Is it right or acceptable (or just part of life) that value judgements come into play when objective measures, such as the MMSE, are being used in routine practice (as opposed to the context of research)?

Even judgements about the efficacy of the medication, therefore, involve a number of evaluative judgements.

Indeed, it was the accounts of family carers which always seemed more convincing than the numbers: 'Mum is remembering the names of her grandchildren more often'; 'He's started helping in the kitchen and laying the table again, which he'd stopped doing'; 'Dad seems more confident again about going out'. Whilst often convincing, these accounts could certainly not always be taken as proof of efficacy, particularly if all sorts of other things had changed during the three months since the drug was started. Perhaps the community psychiatric nurse was now visiting; perhaps the social worker had arranged day care; perhaps the local Alzheimer's Society had organized a befriender. And now Dad was doing better. Often it was convenient to ascribe the improvement to the medication.

Reflection point

We do tend to place value on numbers, but the accounts of family carers and patients themselves are of value; so how do we decide how much weight to put on different accounts of improvement?

It was convenient because the use of the drugs was audited for many years. This was because, at just about £1,000 a year, they were considered expensive. Hence, hearing evidence of improvement was useful for audit purposes. Some of us were annoyed, of course, that £1,000 a year for effective symptomatic treatment of dementia was considered expensive when drugs for a variety of other conditions, from heart disease to cancer, were more expensive but were not surrounded by such bureaucratic monitoring. (We might say this is a good example of someone who 'thinks facts, thinks values' but actually only thinks about values in terms of financial costs!).

Reflection point

What were the values that imposed bureaucratic procedures around the use of cholinesterase inhibitors but not around other, more dangerous drugs? Was this a sign of ageism? NICE guidance still stipulates that a specialist must be involved in the initiation of donepezil. Whose values does this reflect?

In the early days there was another worry. Given that the drug only worked on the acetylcholine between the nerves, and given that the underlying pathology meant the levels of acetylcholine were inexorably declining, at some point it was inevitable that the person would decline back down to the level he or she had reached before. So, what was the benefit in an improvement of a point on the MMSE if it were only to last for six months? Gradually it became apparent that the benefits sometimes persisted. But then a further concern emerged: What if the person's improvement were such as to allow the person insight into the condition? Wouldn't it be terrible for the person who had lost awareness only to regain it and then to realize that this awareness would shortly be lost again? Indeed, we have seen people where this has occurred. Some people have become more distressed on the medication and it is not certain whether this is caused by the drug acting specifically on the brain, in other words as a direct biological side effect, or whether it has reflected a psychosocial side effect, that is, conscious awareness of what is happening. In any event, the distress has often settled when the drug is stopped.

Reflection point

Is it acceptable, even if inevitable, that non-clinical pressures should determine clinical judgement to some extent? If so, how are the values involved in such judgements properly modified?

There was also a situation where a wife, seen as part of a research project, said that the drug had returned her husband to something much more like his former self. But, in fact, she had endured an unhappy marriage with him. He had always been controlling, slightly bullying, and domineering. When he developed dementia his personality changed and he became calmer and more affectionate. The drug had changed him back to his more controlling and mildly aggressive self. She asked the doctors to stop the medication and he became more lovable again.

Reflection point

Who should decide whether the drug is beneficial? What values are suggested by our answers to this question? (Was it right for the wife and GP to stop the drug in order to improve matters for the wife with the erstwhile irritable husband?)

The bureaucratic business of auditing the use of the drugs to show efficacy itself had a distorting effect. In the MMSE, the person has to repeat the sentence 'No ifs, ands, or buts'. What if they missed one or two of the 's' noises, saying 'No ifs and, or buts', should they be given the point? Standardized scoring says it must be exact in order to get the point. But what if this is the point that makes a difference between a definite improvement or not and, hence, the difference between staying on the drug or not? What if, during testing of orientation for time, they seem to be prompted by something or someone, for example, the daughter nodding or smiling at the birthday cards?

Further, if the diagnosis was being made at the person's home and all that was to hand was a copy of a brain scan report which indicated mild ischaemic change and mild atrophy (i.e. some blockages of the small blood vessels and some slight shrinkage of the brain), it might be debatable whether or not this could be called Alzheimer's disease. If the history was in keeping with Alzheimer's, such a scan might be regarded as supportive. But, rightly or wrongly, given that the only positive finding of the scan was of vascular damage (i.e. a problem with the blood flow), it might be said this could instead be labelled vascular dementia. The inclination to make this judgement might be increased by a history of a 'funny turn', which could represent a tiny stroke, or by a history of risk factors such as hypertension (raised blood pressure) or smoking. Funny turns, hypertension, and smoking are not completely uncommon in older people, and not everyone with these factors in their history will have vascular dementia. However, if you are pressed for time and want to avoid filling in pieces of paper to audit your use of the cholinesterase inhibitor, a natural inclination might be to call this vascular dementia, for which the drugs are not licensed. In other words, clinicians sometimes settled for an easy diagnosis of vascular dementia, whereas further investigations might have made an Alzheimer's disease diagnosis the more likely, because this avoided work: the patient did not have to be seen again. The point to notice is that all of the judgements being made here are evaluative and the facts, such as they are, are value-laden.

Reflection point

If people feel too pressured because the system values bureaucratic monitoring very highly, if individual doctors do not value the effects of the drugs as much as others do, if an exact diagnosis is not valued, if services do not place a premium on following up people with vascular dementia, then doctors will be prone to interpret or apply the facts in one way rather than another.

Over the years, there have been changes in the guidance issued by NICE concerning the use of the drugs. The guidance has also been enforced more or less strictly at different times and differently in different parts of the country. Initially, the guidance allowed donepezil and the other cholinesterase inhibitors to be used for mild to moderate Alzheimer's dementia, that is, from a score on the MMSE of 26/30 down to 12/30. But then, in November 2006, NICE evaluated the cost-effectiveness of the drugs and concluded that they should only be used on those with moderate dementia (MMSE scores of 20/30 to 10/30). The drug companies, the Alzheimer's Society, and the relevant professional bodies came together in a storm of protest. The High Court allowed a judicial review on the grounds that NICE's guidance was discriminatory, and on 10 August 2007 the Court ordered NICE to produce a draft amendment to its guidance. The drug company's challenge to NICE was procedural: that NICE had not been fair and transparent. The guidance is now, once again, that donepezil can be used for mild to moderate disease. During this period of uncertainty, however, clinicians used various techniques to argue that their patients were in the moderate category despite higher scores on the MMSE. But some did not: some stuck to the NICE guidance despite their beliefs that it was wrong.

Reflection point

Changes in judgements by NICE, and the fact that a judicial review ruled against them, suggests that NICE's objective guidance is itself value-laden. In particular, the economic models used by NICE to judge cost-effectiveness are not value-free.

Reflection point

Should we value national guidance, or should we value the possibility that, despite national guidance, using our own (evaluative) judgement, medication will (or will appear) to help the person in front of us (Hughes, 2012)?

Nowadays, the worries about the MMSE score have abated. On the basis of the DOMINO-AD study (Howard et al., 2012), which found that patients with moderate or severe Alzheimer's disease continued to benefit from donepezil, both in terms of cognitive function and general functioning, most clinicians continue to give donepezil into the severer stages of the disease. This is despite the drug not being licensed for use in severe dementia. Incidentally, whereas the cost of donepezil was originally about £1,000 a year, at the time of writing (July 2017), since the patents on donepezil expired in 2010 (and shortly afterwards for the other drugs), the cost is only a little over £10.68 per year.

Reflection point

To what extent should the monetary cost of a drug determine its use? Obviously an enormously expensive drug must be monitored if not rationed by a public health system like the NHS. But there may be a cost threshold below which this will not be the case. Evaluative decisions are involved in deciding how much is too much.

Reflection point

Is it acceptable, even if inevitable, that non-clinical pressures should determine clinical judgement to some extent? If so, how are the values involved in such judgements properly modified?

The reality now is that donepezil is prescribed with much less fuss and most people started on the drug remain on it unless there are side effects. It would, indeed, seem odd not to prescribe donepezil (or one of the other anti-dementia drugs) as a routine treatment for anyone who might have Alzheimer's or one of the other dementias where it is known to be effective, such as DLB or mixed vascular and Alzheimer's dementia.

Reflection point

The current reality of dementia care makes it seem as if the use of the drugs is almost a given. This could amount to excessive medicalization, as if all forgetfulness might warrant treatment in old age. There are values attached to such determinations.

Reflection point

The experience of people in connection with taking donepezil is not well researched. There would be methodological difficulties for sure. But it means we do not know enough about how treatment is valued.

One last point to add to the clinician's story is that almost all of the studies that support the use of the cholinesterase inhibitors have been carried out by teams involving physicians who have received funding from drug companies, including the drug companies that produce the cholinesterase inhibitors. This need not be a bad thing – many of the individuals concerned are people of great integrity who will use drug company money to pursue educational or academic ends without compromising their independence. But it is a point to note, in which case, for the sake of transparency, it must be said that one of the present authors (JCH) has also benefited from drug company sponsorship, including from the manufacturers of the cholinesterase inhibitors.

Prodromal Dementia

'Think facts; think values' is relevant to every aspect of the treatment and diagnosis of dementia. Our discussion of the cholinesterase inhibitors makes this point. Now we shall see that the evaluative nature of decisions that surround dementia runs even deeper. It is not solely whether or not a person has the disease or should be treated that are issues requiring evaluative judgements. This can be said of many other conditions as well: hypertension, for example. There is no objective, factual point at which blood pressure is too high in the absence of evaluative judgements about the harm that might arise. Indeed, there have been debates about the merits or otherwise of treating some degrees of hypertension in older people. Very high blood pressure is associated with strokes and heart attacks; very low blood pressure is associated with fainting and falling. So value judgements have to be made: What levels of risk are we willing to accept? Moreover, we might wish to go much further and say that value judgements surround the diagnosis and treatment of almost all conditions. At what point does the occasional wheeze become asthma in need of treatment? At what precise point do dysplastic cells become cancerous? How long do you leave a mole if you're worried about malignant melanoma? Such questions are part and parcel of clinical practice. They reflect the need to 'think facts; think values'.

These days, in the world of dementia evaluative judgements run deeper. For it is now possible to talk of Alzheimer's disease *without dementia*. For some years we have had the notion of mild cognitive impairment (MCI), which suggests a condition in which, for what is termed the amnestic type of MCI (aMCI), there are:

- Subjective complaints about forgetfulness;
- Objective tests to show memory impairment (reflective of age and education);
- Normal general cognitive functions;
- Normal abilities in terms of everyday activities;
- Insufficient criteria for a diagnosis of dementia.

Although MCI has become an accepted term in the nomenclature surrounding dementia, it is problematic in at least two ways. First, conceptually: it is difficult to know to what it refers. It does not refer to a disease, and it does not even refer to a condition that will become a disease, because some people with MCI do not progress to dementia. In a sense, it simply names the syndrome with which the person presents: they have cognitive impairment, but it's mild. In the amnestic form it mainly affects memory, but there are other forms. It does more than this, however, because the name is a decidedly medical one. The person is labelled as having MCI, which leads to the second problem.

MCI is emotionally and socially stigmatizing. People are told they have something. Further, they have something that may progress to dementia. But no one can say what exactly it is that they have or whether what they have will progress. It is a sort of limbo, but one which can have stigmatizing consequences because people with MCI start to be treated differently. The label is not *just* a label. It can be distressing (Corner and Bond, 2006).

The whole of the first issue of *Philosophy, Psychiatry & Psychology* (*PPP*) in 2006 was devoted to MCI. In it, a number of practitioners and thinkers raised issues about the notion of MCI and its implications. Petersen (2006) defended MCI in the issue as a useful and relevant concept; but there were also criticisms. Some years later this special issue of *PPP* on MCI was referred to critically in an anonymous review of a research proposal which sought to consider some of the social determinants of the concept (later the research was published: Moreira et al., 2008). The reviewer, obviously annoyed at the implied criticism of the concept, referred to the issue of *PPP* as having been troublemaking and irresponsible (or words to this effect).

The outburst by the anonymous reviewer might just be regarded as aberrant behaviour. However, the upshot of the research, which was eventually funded, was also vilified in some quarters. All of this might seem bizarre, because it would seem really quite reasonable to suggest that a notion such as MCI raises questions about what is and is not normal. It raises questions about boundaries and, implicitly, about the standing of 'dementia' itself as a medical phenomenon (Hughes, 2011, 2013).

It is indubitably a matter of sociological and ethical interest. It touches on the problem of the medicalization of normal ageing. One manifestation of this is that everything is seen, or couched, in a biomedical light. A concomitant is that people should accept treatment for their medical conditions. Thus, we have seen how cholinesterase inhibitors have become the norm. The drive to early diagnosis, whatever it is (perhaps a means to encourage ACP and good support), is also a drive towards treatment with cholinesterase inhibitors with their modest benefits. It has also become normal for anyone with forgetfulness, but without dementia, to be told they have MCI, as if this is helpful in itself.

Of course, what is interesting about the outburst by the reviewer for our purposes is that it shows how the facts about MCI are not just facts, because 'think facts; think values'. The truth is that the values attached to labels such as MCI are deeply embedded but are also diverse. Our suggestion is that we need to see clearly the evaluative judgements that might be at work. But even this modest suggestion can seem like an affront to those devoted to the cause of MCI.

They would argue that if we are to cure Alzheimer's disease, we need to identify the states that lead to it. If we can pinpoint the type of MCI that leads to Alzheimer's disease, then we are more likely to identify the pathological mechanisms that lead to Alzheimer's, and this brings cure ever closer. If this is the case, then anyone who turns up suggesting that MCI is a sociological phenomenon raising ethical concerns about the medicalization of normal ageing is just a nuisance. The value of medical advance, of curing Alzheimer's disease, might seem so overwhelming that anything or anyone who gets in the way is likely to be regarded as a gadfly – an irritating annoyance to be swatted away. But there are values which are felt strongly by those who question the use or purpose of labels such as MCI. Moreover, the facts that surround MCI *just do* seem to be value-laden. Whether or not, for instance, we regard forgetfulness as something to seek medical help for is a value judgement. For some, what used to be called 'benign senescent forgetfulness' is just that: it's the forgetfulness associated with getting old and it needs no more attention. But MCI is immediately something more sinister, which demands medical attention.

One of the questions being considered at about the time of the *PPP* special issue on MCI was whether, indeed, the cholinesterase inhibitors might be effective in MCI. The suggestion that MCI was a (mere) social construct must then have seemed particularly gadfly-ish to the drug companies trying to find new markets for their drugs. The clash was not particularly a clash of facts, but a clash of values. Subsequently, research has confirmed that cholinesterase inhibitors are not useful in MCI (Russ and Morling, 2012).

The advent of biomarkers – from genetics and cerebrospinal fluid markers to neuroimaging – means that it is now possible to detect Alzheimer's pathology in the brain before dementia has made itself manifest. Hence, as we said before, it is now possible to have a non-dementia form of Alzheimer's disease. This possibility simply raises the evaluative questions that surrounded MCI in a new form. And there are twists. As in the case of MCI, different people will place a different value on having a 'diagnosis', if we can call these presentations 'diseases'. Some people, completely free of any symptoms, so not 'ill' in any sense, would wish to know that they have biomarkers that suggest they might go on to have the disease. What level of certainty should attach to such prognostications will also be a matter of evaluative concern. But some people would not wish to know this news under any circumstances. They would not value such knowledge, especially if it were knowledge with a great deal of uncertainty attached to it.

What if screening programmes were developed? How much pressure would individuals feel under to be screened if, for instance, they had a family history of dementia? One of the accepted preconditions for a screening programme is that there should be some chance of a successful treatment. However, the nature of such success and the nature of the treatment could be debated. So there would be evaluative judgements that provided advice on reducing risks and planning for the future so important that screening would be sanctioned. The pressure for screening would increase if there were new symptomatic treatments. Of course, the pressure for a screening programme would be immense if there were a certain cure. And the pressure would reflect the strength of the shared values. In the absence of a cure, the values are likely to be more diverse.

A different scenario is where researchers are routinely discovering that individuals test positive for the biomarkers of dementia (chiefly Alzheimer's disease). The ethical issue is whether participants in research should be told, especially if there is little to be done, and especially if there is any uncertainty. Again, there will be different answers to questions about disclosure depending on the values held by different people. New discoveries in science, therefore – and as we shall discuss in more detail in the next chapter – are raising new ethical values (Hughes et al., 2017).

'Think facts; think values', therefore, turns out to be highly applicable to the diagnosis, not only of different forms of dementia but also to MCI and other prodromal stages, even many years before the pathology is apparent. One of the key pathological markers, indeed, is amyloid. The exact role of amyloid in the pathogenesis of Alzheimer's disease is not clear. We know that normal older people have amyloid in their bodies – and indeed a variety of other 'pathological' markers. So the whole business of determining at a biological level where true pathology begins is not straightforward. The determinations that are made, therefore, although based on facts, involve values. Dementia and prodromal dementia are fact-full but are value-laden too.

Background Frameworks

So far in this chapter we have been able to show how, in connection with particular aspects of dementia or dementia care, facts and values go together. Before concluding, we want to make the point that this is a general feature of our world. It is part of the framework by which we live. We describe the world in many ways. This will involve many facts of different sorts: the facts of biology, of chemistry, and of physics, as well as the facts of geography and anthropology. But we do not capture the world, even if such a thing were possible, in the absence of values.

Take facts about insects, for instance. The facts that entomologists deal with are just facts in one sense: insects have six legs; the migratory locust, *Locusta migratoria*, shows differences in its aerobic metabolism, which is under genetic control, depending on whether it lives at high altitudes (e.g. the Tibetan Plateau) or low altitudes (e.g. the North China Plain) such that the Tibetan Plateau locusts can tolerate hypoxia better than the North China Plain locusts (Zhao, 2013). Whether simple or complex, facts about insects are value-laden in the broad sense that our knowledge of insects can affect how we live with them. How do we, for instance, deal with swarms of locusts? What value do we place on the harms that follow from the bioaccumulation of pesticides in the food chain? Values around the use of pesticides will be diverse.

On the other hand, the evaluative judgement that we should call all six-legged animals 'insects' is commonly shared. The phylogenetic discovery that there may be some six-legged animals that are not insects, such as flightless springtails (which turn out to be more like hermit crabs than locusts), causes disruption to the shared values base. What we certainly cannot say is that entomology has nothing to do with values.

The broader point is that facts about the world will raise questions, concerns, judgements, disputes, and opinions of an evaluative nature. This is a feature of the complexity of the world. Facts are always seen against a background, and the background almost inevitably contains values. These sorts of background frameworks – the evaluative concerns, opinions, and so on – can be considered scaffolding for our day-to-day activities, and recall that values are action-guiding. In addition, the background can be seen from different perspectives. Thus, the background to the facts about cholinesterase inhibitors is that there are different value judgements about the benefits of cognitive function and about the place of medication in our lives. The background to MCI is seen differently by some scientists and by some sociologists. Perhaps in one case (but this is likely to be an oversimplification) the background involves the onward march of the objective understanding of organic degenerative brain conditions, whereas in the other case the background is that of the onward march towards the broader applicability of theories around social construction and labelling. There are ways in which different backgrounds, or the perception of them, can be brought together. But there are also ways in which they may become entrenched, so that adherents of a particular view can only see this one view and feel belligerent towards alternative views. And such strongly held views invariably reflect trenchant values.

These backgrounds can be called myths. This is not to denigrate them. A myth need not be wholly fictitious, and myths, as stories, provide explanations for the phenomena of life. This topic has been wonderfully considered in Mary Midgley's book *The Myths We Live By*:

> Myths are not lies. Nor are they detached stories. They are imaginative patterns, networks of powerful symbols that suggest particular ways of interpreting the world. They shape its meaning. (Midgley, 2004: 1)

Midgley highlights how 'science' can have different meanings:

> We do indeed sometimes think of science just as an immense store-cupboard of objective facts, unquestionable data about such things as measurements, temperatures and chemical composition. But a store-cupboard is not, in itself, very exciting.
>
> (Midgley, 2004: 3)

She continues:

> What makes science into something much grander and more interesting than this is the huge, ever-changing imaginative structure of ideas by which scientists strive to connect, understand and interpret these facts. (2004)

It is in this grander scheme that values exist, emerge, settle, take root, or cause controversy. One of the ideas to which Midgley refers is that of the physical world, including the human body, working like a machine. This conception emerged in the Enlightenment as a bedrock belief in science. The world, including our bodies, could be understood in mechanistic terms. Midgley points out that sciences, such as physics, have had to give up this picture, or myth, as being too simple. Nevertheless, it persists even in descriptions of how the brain works (or does not work) in dementia.

The model that supports the use of cholinesterase inhibitors can be presented in a purely mechanistic way. Cognitive neuropsychological models, according to which the brain works simply like a computer, employ the same stories to understand dementia. Such stories have their uses (see Hughes, 2011: 131–44), but they can also instil pictures which are not so helpful. The brain as a machine is useful in some respects but can distance us from other (psychosocial) ways of dealing with other aspects of dementia.

An obvious example would be behaviour that is found challenging. For example, the person who has always hitherto been placid becomes aggressive and violent as his or her dementia progresses. One explanation for this is that the dementia has caused an upset in the neurochemicals that govern behaviour in the brain. Hence, on this view, the answer might be to give medication to settle the behaviour. An alternative view is that the behaviour reflects the psychosocial surroundings, and the 'treatment' is to understand the person's psychosocial world. This makes it possible that a different approach, a person-centred one, will ameliorate the behaviour. Which approach we adopt will depend on our worldviews, and our worldviews themselves involve values and evaluative judgements. Indeed, such values might clash in a manner that cannot be settled. Some person-centred practitioners might castigate those who rely on medications that are likely to have harmful side effects and could be life-threatening. Prescribers of medication might view those who adopt a behavioural approach as naïve – a naïvety which could prolong distress and is itself risky in terms of the harm that might be done to or by someone with marked agitation. Of course, it doesn't take too much to see that a mixture of approaches might be beneficial: medication at the lowest possible dose for as short a time as possible whilst a behavioural formulation is developed and a behavioural approach negotiated.

Elsewhere, in her book *Science and Poetry,* Mary Midgley has put matters thus:

> There is no way we can collect facts about any significant aspect of human life without looking at them from some particular angle. We have to guide our selection by means of some value-judgement about what matters in it and what does not. And these judgements inevitably arise out of each enquirer's moral position.

(Midgley, 2001: 147)

If our moral positions themselves entail our values, then it can be seen that – if we are to be realistic about our complex world – it is almost impossible not to think values when we think facts.

Conclusion

In this chapter, we have considered how facts and values always go together:

- Facts and values are partners;
- Values cannot take over from facts: evidence is important and must be taken on its merits, but it is only as good as it can be;
- The importance we attach to particular facts reflects our values and, as such, requires some form of evaluative judgement;
- The interplay of facts and values is evident in our attitude towards MCI and other potential stages of prodromal dementia; and
- Our use of medications, such as the cholinesterase inhibitors, also reflects background values.

Discussing the tensions between facts and values and the importance of seeing them together with a degree of clarity ('think facts; think values'), of seeing them, indeed, not as alternatives but as part of a whole complex way of understanding a complex world, is another way of articulating our overall Manifesto:

- Dementia is not something outside our common humanity; it is part of the complex world which we coinhabit;

- Dementia is a disease, for which evidence is crucial; but it is also a disability surrounded by important social and psychological variables that reflect values and rights;
- VBP is one way in which we can deal with the complexity of dementia; and that is in part by taking values seriously.

References

Alzheimer's Disease International. (2016). *World Alzheimer Report 2016: Improving Healthcare for People Living with Dementia – Coverage, Quality and Costs Now and in the Future.* London: ADI. Available at: www.alz.co.uk/research/WorldAlzheimerReport2016.pdf [last accessed 9 August 2017].

Corner, L., and Bond, J. (2006). The impact of the label of Mild Cognitive Impairment on the individual's sense of self. *Philosophy, Psychiatry, & Psychology,* **13**(1): 3–12.

Howard, R., McShane, R., Lindesay, J., et al. (2012). Donepezil and memantine for moderate-to-severe Alzheimer's disease. *New England Journal of Medicine,* **366**: 893–903. doi: 10.1056/NEJMoa1106668

Hughes, J. C. (2011). *Thinking Through Dementia.* Oxford: Oxford University Press.

(2012). Justice, guidelines, and virtues. In H. Lesser, ed., *Justice for Older People.* Amsterdam and New York: Ropodi, pp. 181–99.

(2013). Dementia is dead, long live ageing: Philosophy and practice in connection with 'dementia'. In K. W. M. Fulford, M. Davies, R. G. T. Gipps, et al., eds., *Oxford Handbook of Philosophy and Psychiatry.* Oxford: Oxford University Press, pp. 835–50.

Hughes, J. C., Ingram, T. A., Jarvis, A., et al. (2017). Consent for the diagnosis of preclinical dementia states: A review. *Maturitas,* **98**: 30–34.

Hughes, J. C., Louw, S. J., and Sabat, S. R., eds. (2006). *Dementia: Mind, Meaning, and the Person.* Oxford: Oxford University Press.

Midgley, M. (2001). *Science and Poetry.* London and New York: Routledge.

(2004). *The Myths We Live By.* London and New York: Routledge.

Moreira, T., Hughes, J. C., Kirkwood, T., et al. (2008). What explains variations in the clinical use of mild cognitive impairment (MCI) as a diagnostic category? *International Psychogeriatrics,* **20**(4), 697–709.

NICE. (2011). *Donepezil, Galantamine, Rivastigmine and Memantine for the Treatment of Alzheimer's Disease. Technology Appraised Guidance.* London: National Institute for Health and Care Excellence. Available at: www.nice.org.uk/guidance/ta217/resources/donepezil-galantamine-rivastigmine-and-memantine-for-the-treatment-of-alzheimers-disease-82600254699973 [last accessed on 9 August 2017].

Petersen, R. C. (2006). Mild Cognitive Impairment is relevant. *Philosophy, Psychiatry, & Psychology,* **13**(1): 45–49.

Russ, T. C., and Morling, J. R. (2012). Cholinesterase inhibitors for mild cognitive impairment. *Cochrane Database Systematic Reviews,* Sep 12;(9): CD009132. doi: 10.1002/14651858.CD009132.pub2

Russell, B. (1967). *The Problems of Philosophy.* Oxford: Oxford University Press.

Zhao, D., Zhang, Z., Cease, A., Harrison, J., and Kang, L. (2013). Efficient utilization of aerobic metabolism helps Tibetan locusts conquer hypoxia. *BMC Genomics,* **14**: 631. doi: 10.1186/1471-2164-14-631

The Science-Driven Principle and Dementia

Chapter

9

Topics covered in this chapter
- How the science-driven principle is evident in dementia care: advances in science and technology do not shut down the evaluative judgements that are required; instead, they increase the scope for value judgements.
- We revisit this issue in connection with the issues around early diagnosis.
- We consider quality-of-life (QoL) research as an example of the search for a scientific answer to a question which ultimately also requires evaluative judgements.
- Artificial feeding is an area where advances in science have increased our choices and thereby tested our values.
- The science of ageing research itself creates value judgements.

Take-away message for practice
It is easy for any of us to be impressed by advances in science and technology. But we must nevertheless be alert to the potential for such advances to disrupt (positively and negatively) our underpinning values.

Introduction

This chapter picks up a point made in the previous chapter about the science-driven principle of VBP. The principle suggests that advances in medical science and technology drive the need for VBP precisely because they present us with new choices. In other words, science and technology have the potential to open up a diversity of values. Rather than new scientific knowledge shutting down discussion, it opens it up precisely because of its tendency to reveal the need to think about values in more depth, afresh, or anew.

To take an obvious example, Einstein's theory of special relativity established the equivalence of mass and energy, which was eventually summed up by the famous equation: $E = mc^2$. This scientific insight led scientists to understand more about the strength of nuclear bonds, and the rest (as they say), from atom bombs to nuclear power plants, is history. But this is decidedly not a case of science shutting down discussion! A few (albeit brilliant) scientific facts have exposed a host of divergent values, from those around the possibility (or not) of nuclear weapons acting as a deterrent, to all the debates about nuclear power as a safe source of energy. Once again, it's never just facts, but always facts *and* values. And the advances of science and technology encourage rather than discourage this realization.

In this chapter, we shall look at how this is obvious in connection with dementia. We shall consider four areas. First, we shall revisit the issue of early diagnosis, already raised in the previous chapter. Second, we shall consider the issue of quality of life. Third, we shall consider the specific example of artificial feeding. Finally, we shall position dementia in the context of ageing more generally.

We also wish to pick up the threads of our Manifesto's basic tenets: that dementia is a unique touchstone for understanding the human condition; that it's both a disease and a disability; and that VBP provides an essential (albeit not the only) framework for providing support, care, and treatment to people with dementia, their families, and friends.

Prodromal Dementia

We discussed in the last chapter how our understanding of dementia has expanded so that we now realize that there is a long period of time, maybe even 20 years, when a person might have the pathology of Alzheimer's disease in his or her brain but no symptoms or signs. (This might also be true of other dementias, such as dementia with Lewy bodies and frontotemporal degeneration, but the research tends to consider Alzheimer's.) The pathology can be demonstrated by brain scans, which can now show the presence of amyloid and tau in the brain. These are both proteins at the heart of the pathology of Alzheimer's – amyloid is in the plaques and tau is in the neurofibrillary tangles that characterize the disease. Genetics and testing of cerebrospinal fluid (CSF) provide other biomarkers which, if positive, make the presence of Alzheimer's pathology more likely. We have already suggested in the previous chapter ways in which the possibility of making the diagnosis of a prodromal state raises ethical issues:

- Should people be told that they have markers which are more or less likely to indicate that they will get dementia later?

Our different responses to this question reflect our different values. The advances in science and technology have opened up new choices and, in so doing, have exposed a diversity of values, just as the science-driven principle of VBP predicts. Thus, VBP becomes more relevant as EBP proceeds.

In order to consider this in a little more detail, we shall look at a particular paper. In a sense, this is silly. It's silly because the authors of the paper certainly would not suggest that their paper was the last word. Apart from anything else, this is not how science works: there is always further work to be done, further facts to be clarified. In addition, fixing on this paper (or any one paper) may be silly because it may be eclipsed and considered of no consequence even before our book has gone into print. Finally, it is a scientific paper, and one of the things that we are going to point out is that it hardly even nods in the direction of values. But, it might be argued, it would be unreasonable to expect it to do so. As a scientific paper, it makes no claims beyond the science. With this view we can have some sympathy (why should a scientist feel compelled to discuss ethics any more than a philosopher feel compelled to discuss science?). It is, however, not an incontrovertible view, and we would like to raise questions about it, questions that are encouraged by VBP.

The paper is chosen as a matter of convenience – it came to our attention at the time of writing. It was published in the journal *Neurobiology of Aging* in 2017. Actually, we don't think it's silly at all to look at this one paper! First, even if the detailed findings of the paper are one day eclipsed, the thrust of the research (to enable earlier diagnosis) is a major research enterprise, so some of the points we make in connection with this paper will be relevant more broadly. Second, the paper is a good one and yet it exemplifies two points: (1) scientific papers rarely acknowledge the ethical or conceptual issues they raise; (2) yet they demonstrate the science-driven principle of VBP, because advances in science will often lead to overt values diversity.

The title suggests its main claim: 'Multivariate analyses of peripheral blood leukocyte transcripts distinguish Alzheimer's, Parkinson's, control, and those at risk of developing Alzheimer's' (Delvaux et al., 2017). The paper, which emanates from Arizona State University, addresses the need for 'a reliable, simple, inexpensive blood test for Alzheimer's disease (AD) suitable for use in a primary care setting'. The abstract continues by stating that this need is 'widely recognized'. The authors note that many papers have been published looking for such a blood test, but none has been replicable. In other words, even when it is thought that a blood test to diagnose Alzheimer's has been found, later experiments have not been able to confirm that the test works.

In this paper, the researchers looked at genetic material in white blood cells (leukocyte transcripts) to pick up Alzheimer's-related markers, which included markers of inflammation and cell stress, amongst other things. Their conclusion was that their data 'constitute proof of principle for the potential of leukocyte transcripts for the detection of AD and AD risk' (p. 236). They continued: 'We assert that the multivariate data presented here indicate that transcripts from peripheral blood leukocytes offer the potential to distinguish early AD from ND [nondemented] controls and from PD [Parkinson's disease]. Our data also indicate a prognostic marker of progression to the clinical stages of AD in unimpaired older adults' (p. 236). They went on to say that larger studies would be required to confirm their findings. But, in brief, they were confident that their findings potentially paved the way for a blood test that might be useful in primary care.

In passing, we might wish to challenge the use of language. Talk of the 'non-demented' suggests that there are others who are the 'demented'. Many people use this terminology without reflection. It is, however, a way to lump together 'the demented' as if they were a homogenous group and one that is labelled in a derogatory manner. The authors could, after all, simply have had 'controls'. That they did not signifies certain sorts of attitudes that reflect certain sorts of values.

One thing to say immediately is that the depth, breadth, and quality of the science involved in this paper are not to be underestimated. In addition, the authors have explicitly acknowledged some of the shortcomings of the paper. This is thorough and impressive scientific work. It may well represent, even if only in an embryonic form, a breakthrough that will revolutionize the assessment of people at risk of Alzheimer's disease. But let's now consider whether this is the type of scientific and technological advance that, in keeping with the science-driven principle, might open up choices in a way that reflects and shows a diversity of values.

First, we should go back to the opening of the abstract, which talked about a 'widely recognized' need for a simple blood test. Well, we might wish to question how 'widely recognized' it is that we need to have a simple, reliable, inexpensive blood test for Alzheimer's disease. We should note that, in an otherwise factual scientific paper, this little phrase introduces at least one evaluative judgement. There is no evidence presented, no facts to support the claim, except rather indirectly. Of course, a lot of effort has gone into looking for a reliable test for Alzheimer's, and a simple and cheap one would be better than a complex and expensive one. In addition, researchers have looked at blood tests before. It seems highly likely, therefore, that the research community people would welcome such a test.

But it's not obvious that the research community would widely recognize a blood test to be the best way to achieve an early diagnosis. Being human, it could be that other researchers are more committed to their own technologies – neuroimaging, for example. The point is that researchers themselves might well place different emphases on the usefulness of one diagnostic approach over another. This is likely to be because they value some things rather than others. Some might feel that certainty comes from seeing the pathology of Alzheimer's disease on a brain scan. Science does, of course, provide a way out of any bickering there might be between scientists: it's always possible to do the experiment and to compare diagnosis by blood test and by neuroimaging and see which is better, in the sense of more accurate as well as cheaper, more convenient, and so forth. Even then, differences in terms of values might emerge: How are we going to judge, for instance, what is 'more convenient'? How much weight do we place on the convenience to the person undergoing the tests as opposed to the convenience of the staff?

But we still haven't considered the views of others outside the research community. How 'widely recognized' is the need for a simple, reliable, and inexpensive blood test for Alzheimer's amongst ordinary general practitioners (GPs) or family doctors? Would they all be confident about when to use the test? Would they want the full responsibility of making such a diagnosis to fall squarely on their shoulders? Again, some GPs would relish the opportunity to be able to do such a test themselves; but some would not. These differences would reflect different values. Some may not value early diagnosis in the absence of a cure or treatment that is no more than modest in its effects. Some might just feel that the responsibility for a diagnosis with such serious and complex repercussions should be made in secondary and not primary care. Education might help to change some of these values, but such education will itself reflect values of one sort or another. And there again, we have not yet considered how 'widely recognized' the need for such a test is amongst ordinary people at risk of dementia.

In saying all of this we are making two points. First, the rare interjection of a value judgement into an otherwise rigorous scientific paper lacks a sound evidence base; and, second, it turns out to be at least a little controversial. This is not simply a detail. For the whole paper is based, in a sense, on the foundational statement that it is 'widely recognized' that such a blood test is required. The authors' work does not, of course, depend on this wide recognition of the problem. They could just state that *they* have recognized the need for the blood test and that is why they are publishing the results of their experiment. Implicitly, however, an evaluative judgement has been made.

Landing on the use of the words 'widely recognized' is not peripheral to the bigger point we are making. But let's pause to consider one of its scientific details in order to arrive at that bigger picture. An issue for this blood test to do with its reliability is whether or not it can distinguish between Alzheimer's disease and Parkinson's disease. Even if the tests can distinguish between people living with Alzheimer's disease and people who are not, it could be that the measures for Alzheimer's disease (AD) are picking up people with other neurodegenerative diseases, such as Parkinson's disease. It is important to make sure this is not the case. The findings of the paper, however, show a fair degree of overlap between AD and Parkinson's disease (PD). The text explains that there was 80–85 per cent correctness in distinguishing between the AD and PD groups, which each only had ten people in them. Nevertheless, this was enough to provide statistically significant differences between the two groups. Hence, on this basis, the authors conclude: 'These data are consistent with a suggestion that our results are not detecting a general neurodegenerative phenomenon but do indicate specificity to AD' (p. 232).

Still, we can ask how much the statistical significance means to ordinary people. We are not making the point that most of us do not understand statistics! What we want to ask is:

How reassured would you be if you were told that you were having a test where there was a 15 to 20 per cent chance that the result would be wrong but that statistical analysis had said that the test was good?

We suspect that this would depend on a number of things. After all, 80–85 per cent correctness is not to be sneezed at. But if the consequence of a misdiagnosis were that you would be given the wrong medication, you might not be too happy. It depends on what you value most.

Your views of the blood test would be affected by your views of these sorts of data. The broader point is that our attitudes to blood tests such as these are affected by all sorts of values. Moreover, some of these values are not even apparent until the science has been done to support the new technology. This paper, let alone any subsequent development of a blood test for routine practice, therefore creates choices and potentially reveals a diverse array of values. VBP comes into its own where there is this sort of uncertainty and the need for careful deliberation. Science drives the need for greater VBP. You can check this for yourself by asking the following questions and deciding whether you and your colleagues would have the same answers. In answering these questions, you have to keep in mind that they would only be pertinent in a situation where you had *no symptoms or signs* of dementia.

- If there were a routine blood test for Alzheimer's disease (i.e. for the underlying pathology but in the absence of symptoms or signs) which could be performed by your GP, would you want to have the test?
- Would you want it when you are 40 years old?
- Would you want it when you are 60 years old?
- Would you want it if you had a family history of dementia?
- Would you want it if you did not have a family history of dementia?
- If you drive a car, would you want the test?
- If your main income came from driving, would you want the test?
- Would you want the test as part of a 'routine' medical for a new job?
- Would you want the test if you were applying for a new mortgage?
- If you had the test and it were positive, what would you do?
- If it were positive, would you tell your spouse or partner?
- Would you tell your children if the test were positive?
- Would you tell work colleagues and your manager?
- What would be the effect on you if the results were positive?
- What would be the effect on your family?

New science and new technologies seem obviously to create choices with the possibility of diverse values appearing. The science-driven principle is as relevant to dementia as it is to other branches of science.

But just to go back a little bit, at the start of this section we asked: Why should a scientist feel compelled to discuss ethics any more than a philosopher feel compelled to discuss science? There are good reasons for this: science and scientific papers must be clear and cannot be too speculative. The point of the paper is to say why the experiment was done, how it was done, and what it showed. Nonetheless, there is usually a discussion section in a scientific paper. And, actually, if a philosopher were discussing the implications of Einstein's work, he or she should show some awareness of what Einstein wrote. There would at least have to be a summary of the aspect of the science that was pertinent to the philosophical discussion. Similarly, if a philosopher were writing a paper that raised an issue concerning which science might provide an answer, it would seem remiss not to mention the science. We end this section, therefore, with a question:

Might it not seem reasonable to expect scientists writing in ethically or philosophically controversial areas at least to acknowledge that there is controversy?

Our worry is that in the present context scientists usually do not seem to recognize that different values might be at play. The need for VBP in dementia is clear, as stated in the third of our Manifesto principles:

VBM provides an essential framework for the support, care, and treatment of people with dementia, their family, and their friends.

Quality of Life

It makes perfect sense that we should think about quality of life in connection with dementia. In particular, it makes sense that quality of life should be considered in connection with any interventions. If we do something for people with dementia, from giving a new tablet to arranging a new support service, it makes sense to ask whether it has improved the person's life overall – and by this we mean the person's quality of life. Indeed, thinking about quality of life can be seen as an advance in our thinking. Previously the focus was on cognitive testing, especially memory. A person was given tests of memory before and after a new treatment. With more sophistication, testing extended to include affect, with specific test of mood, and so on. But quality of life has always been seen as a fundamental concern. Whatever all the other scores have suggested, has the person's overall quality of life improved?

This led researchers to start to develop tests for quality of life (QoL). The development of such scales is a complex matter requiring clear thought and understanding. A lot of scientific effort has been put into the development of scales (of any sort) in order to improve their psychometric properties, in particular, their statistical validity and reliability. Validity refers to their ability to measure what they are supposed to measure, but there are then all sorts of criteria against which validity can itself be determined. Reliability is the ability of the test to measure whatever it is supposed to measure consistently. Again, there are different types, for example, depending on whether you are looking for consistency between different people doing the test or consistency over time when the same person performs the test. The psychological measurement of QoL, which is what the psychometrics of QoL scales is all about, is a thoroughly scientific enterprise. Does it show the science-driven principle of VBP at work?

A systematic review of QoL scales in dementia published in 2015 found 126 relevant articles (having screened 6,806 citations) relating to 16 QoL scales (Bowling et al., 2015).

The earliest of the scales was published in 1989 and the latest in 2007. Three were published in 1999, and although three were also published in 2007, the sense is that for a short while QoL in dementia was a research industry, with interest in the topic building during the 1990s, reaching a peak at around the turn of the century, and then diminishing. It certainly feels now as if researchers are, for the most part, content to use one or another of these established measures. (We are deliberately not considering the specific measures individually, partly because this is not a review of the topic – for which readers should consult e.g. Bowling et al., 2015, but also because we would then feel compelled to say why we were discussing one QoL measure rather than another!)

As with so many systematic reviews of the evidence-based literature, the Bowling paper ended up being critical of the evidence. The authors were unable to commend any particular QoL measure. For example, in their abstract they say: 'All measures were tested on selective samples only ... in a few sites. Their general applicability remains unknown, and predictive validity remains largely untested' (Bowling et al., 2015). Perhaps this should be no surprise because of two inherent problems connected to QoL: the problem of domains and the subjective-objective problem (Hughes and Baldwin, 2006: 96–99).

The *problem of domains* relates to validity. In devising a QoL measure, decisions have to be made about which aspects of life go to make up quality of life. These are the domains. As they discussed each measure in their review, Bowling et al. (2015) listed a variety of items that constituted domains or were constituents of domains (see Box 9.1).

This list does not contain all of the domains, or items from the domains, that exist in the 16 dementia QoL scales reviewed. If it did, it would go on for ever. In one scale there were 27 items in 19 domains; in another there were 53 items; in another, 31 items in 6 domains; and so on. No scale includes all of the items or a definitive set of domains. Some instruments focus on health-related aspects of quality of life. Some take a broader psychological or social view. Even in the list in Box 9.1 it would be reasonable to ask if 'Health' means physical or mental health; or whether 'Function' refers to physical or mental functioning. Box 9.1 could be expanded in a variety of ways. Some measures have been constructed on the basis of expert opinion, some by talking with patients and carers. But the real point is this:

The number of items and domains cannot be pinned down by some sort of experimental process.

The notion of quality of life is inherently uncircumscribable. It is always open to any of us to come up with something new that contributes to our quality of life. It is a notion that cannot be pinned down (Hughes, 2003).

The *subjective-objective* problem contributes to the domain problem, for QoL can be measured either subjectively or objectively. We can ask someone to tell us about their quality of life, or we can observe them and make a decision according to our observations. The difficulty here is that judgements from the outside are notoriously wrong. Others are prone to ascribe a lower quality of life to people with disabilities than those people are to themselves. More sinisterly, sometimes others judge that people with disabilities have no quality of life and that, in fact, their lives are not worth living. This can also be said of people living with dementia. Such statements tend, however, to underestimate the extent to which the social and psychological environment might contribute to the person's quality of life. The nature of the inner or subjective assessment of QoL in dementia, coupled with

Box 9.1 Aspects or Domains of Quality of Life

Daily activities	Social confidence
Looking after self	Hope
Health	Function
Well-being	Leisure
Cognitive functioning	Sleep
Social relationships	Energy
Self-concept	Mobility
Smiling	Environment
Sadness	Mood or affect
Crying	Need-fulfilment
Discomfort	Identity
Irritability	Meeting someone new
Calmness	Making friends
Behavioural signs of comfort	Looking at the stars or moon
Engagement	Spiritual
Eating	Intellectual
Sense of personal growth	Vocational
Sense of agency	

(from Bowling et al., 2015, with permission from Taylor & Francis)

the problem of domains, means that it cannot in the end be measured in any definitive manner (Hughes, 2003).

Nevertheless, failing to notice the implications of such conceptual problems, Bowling et al. (2015) bravely conclude their review by saying: 'The lack of consensus on measuring QoL in dementia suggests a need for a broader, more rigorously tested QoL measure'. They emphasize the importance of talking with people with dementia themselves. But they don't see that although it is possible to measure all sorts of aspects of QoL, it is not sensible to say that you've got it pinned down.

To return to our theme, one way to see what all of this reveals is to look at it from the perspective of the science-driven principle of VBP. As QoL research has progressed, it has become increasingly obvious that value judgements are required. Which domains shall we measure? What items shall we include in the domains? And over time the evaluative judgements have increased rather than decreased. Scientific thinking and investigation – involving people with dementia, for instance – have broadened the values that are in play in connection with QoL in dementia.

A very reasonable suggestion, therefore, which draws on the third principle of our Manifesto, is that VBP provides an important framework for understanding QoL in dementia. If we are contemplating a study that will affect QoL in dementia, we might wish to consider putting to work aspects of VBP, by recognizing that different people value things differently, by putting the values of the person living with dementia centre stage, by attending to the implied values of the person, by working in partnership with them, by communicating with empathy and subtlety, by hearing the views of all concerned, by negotiating differences, and so on. Measures of QoL should be person-centred and individual to the particular person. He or she should decide whether his or her quality of life has improved or not. Where the person would find it difficult or impossible to convey this information, consultation to assess this should be broad. One observer will not be enough; rather, a variety of observations should be considered, both from professionals from various backgrounds and from those who know the person well. If a particular QoL scale is to be used, it should be acknowledged that it is a partial measure, an indication of QoL in a circumscribed fashion.

In an even stronger sense, issues around QoL in dementia speak to our second Manifesto principle: dementia as disease and disability. Similar issues to do with domains and the subjective-objective problem arise in other forms of disability. But the point is that many people living with other forms of disability have not hesitated to assert their rights. Typically, such rights do not reflect the rights of groups as such, but of individuals: individual human rights. People with dementia in most situations do not wish to be judged as a group. There is a slogan, attributed to the late Tom Kitwood, that once you've met one person with dementia, you've met *only* one person with dementia. The quality of life of one person with dementia may depend on very different things in comparison with that of another. The best QoL measures have been constructed with input from people living with dementia. Even so, they have mostly been used and then not referred to again. They've supplied their data anonymously and moved on. Contrariwise, the only really valid measure of QoL is the estimation of the person in conjunction with a discussion with the person and with his or her carers, as seems most appropriate: domains will thus be personal, and skilled interviewing may allow the subjective-objective problem to be negotiated for the individual. This would be to honour the rights and dignity of the person living with dementia as disability. Of course, such an approach seems very impractical, so researchers must find ways of approximating. But what they must not do is think they have captured QoL for all people living with dementia.

Artificial Feeding

Attempts to feed people artificially, when they are not able to eat and swallow normally, have probably been pursued for hundreds of years. Surgical interventions to allow food to be placed directly into the stomach were increasingly attempted in the 1800s. But percutaneous endoscopic gastrostomy (PEG) was devised as a technique in 1979, when a paediatric surgeon, M. W. L. Gauderer, and a gastroenterologist, J. L. Ponsky, performed surgery on a six-month-old child in Cleveland, Ohio (Minard, 2006).

The technique is performed using an endoscope (a thin flexible tube with a light that can be used to see inside the stomach) to place a feeding tube (the PEG tube) through the surgically created hole (the gastrostomy) that links the skin of the abdominal wall to the stomach. There are risks to the procedure (such as infection or haemorrhage) and, indeed, people can die as a result. But on the whole, PEG tubes can be inserted without too many problems into people who are quite frail, and they are easier in some ways than tubes through the nose (nasogastric tubes), which people are more prone to pull out. People live for years being fed by a PEG tube. Giving nutrition into veins (parenteral nutrition) is even more precarious than trying to use a nasogastric tube, because of the risk of infection, and is not generally considered feasible as a long-term means of feeding someone.

Vignette - Mr Almeida: To feed or not to feed?

Mr Almeida had received a diagnosis of mixed Alzheimer's and vascular dementia about ten years ago. For the last three years he had been totally dependent on staff in his nursing home for all of his needs. He was unable to speak any longer, was incontinent, and had to be changed and repositioned to avoid pressure sores. He had also developed swallowing problems. He was seen by the speech and language therapist, who gave advice to the staff about using thickened fluids and demonstrated the correct posture for Mr Almeida to be fed. This worked for a while, but the process of feeding Mr Almeida was time-consuming.

Gradually, over time, even when fed correctly, using all of the tips provided by the speech and language therapist, it became obvious that Mr Almeida was choking more often, with frequent coughing fits whilst he was being fed. These episodes of choking could be upsetting for the staff, as they were for Mr Almeida himself and for his family. They became particularly bad after he seemed to have a 'funny turn'. He was not able to swallow anything without choking and the episodes of choking lasted longer. He developed a chest infection. This time, when the speech and language therapist was asked to review Mr Almeida, the opinion given was that it would no longer to be safe to feed him by mouth.

Three options were considered. First, some in the team felt that feeding by a PEG tube would now be in order. Second, given his frail state, there were some people involved in his care who felt that he should be left to slip away. However, the third option of feeding him small amounts very carefully by spoon, whilst accepting the possibility that he might aspirate – that is, that food might get into his lungs with the risk of a major infection – seemed ethically reasonable.

From the perspective of the science-driven principle, the use of PEG tubes to feed people with severe dementia artificially is a case in point. Before PEG tubes, the choices facing those concerned with the care of someone like Mr Almeida were limited. There was no good method of artificial feeding; PEG feeding provides such a method. Prior to PEG tube feeding, people could not be guaranteed appropriate nutrition, so they would fall ill and die. Either they were fed and aspiration pneumonia followed (i.e. a chest infection caused by food entering the trachea and getting into the lungs); or they were not fed and died from inanition (i.e. exhaustion caused by lack of nourishment). PEG feeding increases the options. Indeed, it does more than this: it seems to promise there will be no more problems with feeding.

Sadly, this is not the case. The relevant facts are that PEG feeding does not achieve many of the things that it promises. People can still aspirate. Weight does not always increase. In short, there is no evidence that PEG feeding is of benefit for people with severe dementia (Sampson et al., 2009). But, as they often say, the absence of evidence is not evidence of absence! In other words, it may just be hard to collect the sort of evidence that would count. Some people seem to do well with PEG tubes. Historically, they have often been used in the United States, even if their use is lower in the UK and other European countries. So not everyone would be against the first option of inserting a PEG tube to feed Mr Almeida. Those who encourage a palliative approach, or who instinctively shy away from medical interventions, might go for the second option and argue that he should be allowed to slip away. But others might object that this is too negative and is a form of passive euthanasia, which should be opposed. The third option, to continue feeding in a pragmatic fashion, might seem like a derogation of duty to the frail when there is a potential means to stop further suffering by the insertion of a simple PEG feeding tube.

What we see, therefore, is the potential for clashes of divergent values. As predicted by the science-driven principle of VBP, a scientific and technological advance has increased choice, but also increased the diversity of values at play. Notably in this case, we see this at the personal level and at a societal level. It may be that two professionals would disagree about what is best for Mr Almeida. It may be that the family would hold different views from each other, or from the professional view. But it may also be that a psychiatrist and gastroenterologist in the UK would have different views when compared with a psychiatrist and gastroenterologist in the United States. And VBP, in line with the third principle of our Manifesto, offers a process which should be helpful:

VBP provides an essential framework for the support, care, and treatment of people with dementia, their family, and their friends.

Let's consider how this might work for Mr Almeida. The premise is that those involved would show each other mutual respect and respect, in particular, for any differences in values. Staff would need to be aware of and understand the different views of people and the values that underpin those views. Using good communication skills, they would explore these views and use their reasoning abilities to clarify positions. Practice would be person-centred, taking into account Mr Almeida's values and beliefs, putting these centre stage insofar as they are known, and insofar as possible. But this would be in the context of the multidisciplinary team, where everyone felt able to contribute their views from their different expert positions, which would include the positions of the family. Both facts and values would be put on the table. Areas of difference would be made apparent. Through good partnerships and negotiation, showing mutual respect, the point would be to arrive at a balanced decision within a framework of shared values.

This is an idealized view ignoring the bumps and blocks to smooth practice. But it is no more than an idealized view of the sort of process that many teams will go through every day within different contexts. And it's a view that is not too far from reality in many circumstances. It may be a more or less overt process. Where values differ greatly, the process is likely to be bumpier. But it is nevertheless the only process that makes sense in such a situation, unless we are to ride roughshod over someone's values. We'll say more about PEG feeding in Chapter 11.

Ageing Science

There is a very plausible view that the diseases of old age will never be fully understood and, hence, will not be cured until we have understood ageing itself. Thus, heart failure, arthritis, many cancers, and dementia itself, as well as other conditions that are associated with getting older, require an understanding of the ageing process. To put this another way, it can be said that we all age, but we age in different ways. In some, the ageing process will show itself first in terms of arthritic joints; in some men there will be prostate problems and perhaps prostate cancer; the average age for the onset of ovarian cancer in women is about 63; heart and lung problems tend to develop in older people. So the suggestion is, whatever the specific pathology, it might be a better bet to try to treat the general underlying mechanism that constitutes ageing, given that it is the ageing that seems to make the heart, or joint, or whatever, prone to the disease.

All of this might be applied to dementia as well. We can say that the brain ages, but it ages in different ways. In some the pathology that predominates is vascular (i.e. damage to blood vessels). In others, Alzheimer's appears. But many older brains, when examined microscopically after death, reveal a mixture of pathologies. What is it in the ageing process that allows these different pathologies to appear?

This is not a question we are able to pursue. Current trials of the drug metformin, however, which is normally used to treat diabetes, are causing excitement in the world of ageing research. Metformin is known to affect several metabolic and cellular processes associated with ageing. The claim is that if the drug slows ageing, it would potentially slow the onset of a host of other age-related diseases, including dementia.

But, once again, the possibility of anti-ageing treatments shows the science-driven principle at work. Because any discussion of treating ageing *itself* will raise all sorts of controversies, which in turn raise or reveal different evaluative judgements (Nuffield Council on Bioethics, 2018). What is the point of living longer? Is it worth living longer if the quality of life is not going to be good? Can we get quantity and quality? Does this whole endeavour represent scientists playing with fundamental aspects of our lives that should be left alone? Is a lifespan of three score years and ten perhaps enough? Some people will value an extension of life at any cost. Others will value the lives we already have and will not see any point in trying to extend them. Some will place high store on the possibility that defeating ageing will inevitably mean that we live longer and better lives. Others will lump together those who wish to extend longevity and those who wish to live forever and write them off as foolish utopian extremists.

There are some good reasons to bring together ageing and dementia research. Some of these reasons, as outlined earlier, are good biological reasons. But there are other reasons too. Putting dementia into the broader field of ageing allows us to get away from some of the socially stigmatizing attitudes to dementia (albeit there is prejudice against older people generally). It allows us to see the ageing brain as one other manifestation of ageing. Dementia becomes just another condition to be dealt with, rather than something to be shunned. Part of the way to deal with it is to see that dementia is not one condition. This in itself requires that value judgements are made about where we draw lines around different types of dementia, and, indeed, that evaluative decisions must be made about where dementia begins. As the second principle of our Manifesto suggests, understanding dementia as a disability that may arise as one grows older, as well as a disease of ageing, can enable us to draw upon a wide range of values in considering how we support people with dementia.

In any case, '"[d]ementia" is part of ageing and ageing is part of life; but it is our life lived as human beings amongst others' (Hughes, 2013: 847). It is the context of others that means there is likely to be values diversity and VBP comes into its own. But the context of ageing is also a way to take us back to the first principle of the Manifesto:

Dementia is a unique touchstone for understanding the human condition.

We have to face our ageing, which will include dementia for many people, and how we do this will define us as people, as families, and as societies.

Conclusion

The science-driven principle is no less true in the field of dementia than it is in other scientific and technological areas. Science and technology move forward. Genetic research offers the possibility of personalized or precision medicine, but the decisions that result will still require a careful exploration of values. Neuroimaging reveals in ever greater detail the pathophysiology of neurodegenerative conditions such as dementia. But even the most accurate diagnosis does not preclude the possibility of values diversity. And this is relevant to our second Manifesto principle, which stresses that yes, dementia is a disease, but also a disabling condition with which people with the right support should be able to live well. Nevertheless, this requires an assertion of rights: the rights of people living with disability to equal treatment and to equality of standing as citizens. The science-driven principle makes the point that whatever advances are made from the perspective of dementia as a disease, the requirement that we see the person as someone living with a disability and with all the rights that are inherent to this person remains open:

Dementia as a disability emphasizes the rights of people living with dementia to all the normal benefits of citizenship.

Even if we look at the 'soft' end of science, at the great strides that have been made in the social sciences in relation to dementia, the science-driven principle is still pertinent. We can understand more and more about the qualitative aspects of care, but this in itself raises evaluative judgements. How do we make judgements for other people? How do we know what they really want or need? How do we involve them in decisions about them? Hence, we have seen that:

- Specific advances, from diagnosis to PEG feeding to aspects of day-to-day care, increase our choices and make it likely that values diversity results or, at least, that more thought has to be given to values;
- VBP provides a process, based on mutual respect for differing values, by which it is possible to arrive at balanced decisions within a framework of shared values.

Both of these points are in keeping with the third principle of our Manifesto:

VBM provides an essential framework for the support, care, and treatment of people with dementia, their family, and their friends.

But, meanwhile, in revealing to us the importance of values in connection with empirical facts and advances in science and technology, dementia is simply epitomizing the human condition – the first of our Manifesto's principles – as we have just seen. It does this in a unique way, because dementia, perhaps more than other conditions, touches upon features which are central to our lives as human beings. It touches upon our standing as persons, our identity, our selfhood, our ability to make autonomous decisions, our dependence, our interconnectivity, our situated nature as beings in the world. Applied to dementia, the science-driven principle of VBP raises issues that are pertinent to our basic understanding of ourselves. What is a disease? How do we draw lines around what is normal? What is it that adds quality to our lives? How do we make decisions in the face of incapacity or incompetence? How do we age and what is it to age well when faced by the diseases of old age? Thus, and in many more ways:

Dementia is a unique touchstone for understanding the human condition.

References

Bowling, A., Rowe, G., Adams, S., et al. (2015). Quality of life in dementia: A systematically conducted narrative review of dementia-specific measurement scales. *Aging & Mental Health*, **19**: 13–31. http://dx.doi.org/10.1080/13607863.2014.915923

Delvaux, E., Mastroeni, D., Nolz, J., et al. (2017). Multivariate analyses of peripheral blood leukocyte transcripts distinguish Alzheimer's, Parkinson's, control, and those at risk of developing Alzheimer's. *Neurobiology of Aging*, **58**: 225–37. http://dx.doi.org/10.1016/j.neurobiolaging.2017.05.012

Hughes, J. C. (2003). Quality of life in dementia: An ethical and philosophical perspective. *Expert Review of Pharmacoeconomics and Outcomes Research*, 3, 525–34.

(2013). Dementia is dead, long live ageing: Philosophy and practice in connection with "dementia". In: *Oxford Handbook of Philosophy and Psychiatry* (eds. K. W. M. Fulford, M. Davies, R. G. T. Gipps, et al.); pp. 835–50. Oxford: Oxford University Press.

Hughes, J. C., and Baldwin, C. (2006). *Ethical Issues in Dementia Care: Making Difficult Decisions*. London and Philadelphia: Jessica Kingsley.

Minard, G. (2006). The history of surgically placed feeding tubes. *Nutrition in Clinical Practice*, 21, 626–33.

Nuffield Council on Bioethics. (2018). *Bioethics Briefing Note: The Search for a Treatment for Ageing*. London: Nuffield Council on Bioethics. Available via: http://nuffieldbioethics.org/wp-content/uploads/The-search-for-a-treatment-for-ageing-FINAL-online.pdf (last accessed 28 January 2018).

Sampson, E. L., Candy, B., and Jones, L. (2009). Enteral tube feeding for older people with advanced dementia. *Cochrane Database of Systematic Reviews*, Issue 2. Art. No.: CD007209. http://dx.doi.org/10.1002/14651858.CD007209.pub2

Chapter 10

The Squeaky Wheel Principle

Topics covered in this chapter

- This chapter considers issues around diagnosis and the acceptance of the diagnosis in order to illustrate areas where conflicting values cause noise, often because there is not enough evidence to oil disputes and disagreements.
- There are considerable uncertainties in dementia care, and the impact of a diagnosis can be different in different social and cultural contexts.
- Facts and values can become enmeshed in dementia, as in other areas of our lives, which is seen clearly in relation to rights.
- Rights appear concrete and factual in some lights, but they reflect values; and in other lights rights can seem less important than the values that underpin them.

Take-away message for practice

Sometimes values will rightly dominate, because the evidence is not robust enough to provide us with good quality evidence; even so, as facts emerge, they should be used to check and refine our decisions.

Introduction

The 'squeaky wheel' principle in values-based practice (VBP) is based on the idea that problems involving values often have a way of drawing attention to themselves and this requires a considered response, but it's also important not to lose sight of evidence and facts when these situations arise. When values are 'squeaking' they may need 'lubrication' through the application of VBP, but using evidence and facts can also be helpful. Just as Chapter 8 emphasized the notion of 'think facts; think values', so this chapter makes the point that it is equally as important to 'think values; think facts' too!

Yet, as we have discussed, it's clear that there are a number of potential squeaky wheels that dementia can cause, as well as a limited evidence base to draw upon in many aspects of dementia care. This chapter considers the key areas where squeaky wheels may arise and partly focuses on the diagnosis and acceptance of dementia. This is a crucial area of dementia practice and helps illustrate the three key principles of our Manifesto. But sometimes the dividing line between facts and values in a situation involving a person with dementia isn't always clear, because there are key factors in play which seem to involve elements of both. Different levels of awareness, knowledge, or understanding involving a blurring of facts and values also create squeaky wheels. The way facts and values may be multi-faceted is exemplified by the concept of rights. Thus, this chapter also considers how VBP can work alongside a rights-based approach and assist in situations where values are not the sole cause of squeaky wheels.

Squeaky Wheels Are Everywhere

Experiencing disagreements where people have different values is part of life, irrespective of whether or not one has dementia. Disagreements may involve deeply held beliefs, but they may also occur where facts or evidence can support different viewpoints – listen to how some politicians argue! Where there is irrefutable proof or evidence supporting a position, it's harder to disagree based upon values alone (though people with strong beliefs – as seen in some religious or political arguments – sometimes try to do so). So values tend to draw attention to themselves and create problems – squeaky wheels – where there is limited or conflicting evidence. But that doesn't mean we should ignore the evidence that does exist. In this respect, the squeaky wheel principle is part of everyday life and at work in the multiplicity of interactions between individuals, groups, communities, and societies. The connection between the first element of our Manifesto – 'dementia as humanity' – and the squeaky wheel principle is therefore very clear.

Squeaky Wheels in Dementia

It could be argued that for many years dementia was the squeaky wheel of health care in countries where it was prevalent. As populations of older people have grown, so the impact of dementia has become more apparent, and increasing concern has been expressed about the very limited medical or policy solutions. In the UK, for example, media stories and public reports about poor dementia care over the last 15–20 years represent societal expression of values about existing policy and service responses not being good enough: something had to be done. The squeaky wheel had become deafening, and policy makers responded, partly by looking for what available evidence existed to develop new strategies and services (Department of Health, 2009). The same period also witnessed new or reformed national and international legal frameworks being implemented in the UK and elsewhere affecting dementia care and adding different squeaks to the wheel with which practitioners found themselves grappling (see Chapter 2).

Where there is limited evidence, or a consensus of values is lacking concerning a particular health condition, a wide range of values may become apparent in how a person experiences and expresses the condition, and how carers and practitioners understand and respond to the condition. This creates lots of potential situations which may result in disagreements or misunderstandings – more squeaky wheels. As we have seen, this is frequently the case in many aspects of dementia care, but it is worth reminding ourselves of some of the main areas where this can occur.

The Different Forms of Dementia and the Variation in Their Symptoms

While knowledge has increased significantly about the different forms of dementia, it is still closely linked to the loss of memory and cognitive function associated with Alzheimer's disease. Yet it is estimated that Alzheimer's disease accounts for 62 per cent, (i.e. less than two-thirds) of people with dementia in the UK (Prince et al., 2014). Many dementias are of mixed origin (i.e. they involve more than one type, often Alzheimer's and vascular dementia), but the exact prevalence of mixed dementia is debated, depending on how it has been diagnosed. Zekry et al. (2002) report that neuropathological studies give a prevalence range of between 0 and 55 per cent, but they suggest that the true prevalence might be between 20 and 40 per cent. Less common forms of dementia (e.g. dementia with Lewy bodies [DLB], frontotemporal dementia, Parkinson's dementia) are said to account for another 11 per cent (Fratiglioni et al., 1999). In fact, DLB accounts for just under 20 per cent of all cases of dementia seen at autopsy (McKeith et al., 2005), suggesting that it is underdiagnosed during the lifetime. Different types of dementia can involve quite different symptoms (e.g. hallucinations, disinhibited or uncharacteristic behaviour). The prevalence of psychotic symptoms (hallucinations and delusions) in Alzheimer's disease is anywhere between 10 and 73 per cent, with most studies putting the range at between 28 and 38 per cent (Corey-Bloom and Rafii, 2017). In DLB, visual hallucinations are evident in 33 per cent of people at the time of diagnosis, but the range is from 11 to 64 per cent; and visual hallucinations occur at some point in the course of DLB in 46 per cent, with a range (in different studies) of between 13 and 80 per cent (McKeith, 2017). In one large prevalence study of Alzheimer's disease, anxiety and depression were found in about 37 per cent of people (Aalten et al., 2007). Depression is also very common in vascular and other types of dementia, and large numbers of people living with dementia also experience co-morbidities with physical health conditions.

A lack of clarity about symptoms, confusion caused by multiple symptoms, lack of knowledge, and misunderstandings about different forms of dementia may all result in carers or practitioners responding according to different beliefs and values. The person with dementia, meanwhile, may attribute the effects of dementia to another health condition, such as depression, and deny they have dementia. The subjective experience of dementia, self-understanding, and the complex interactions between individuals mean that the wheel may well squeak. But it's important to recognize that there is still a body of evidence about the different forms of dementia to be drawn upon.

The Causes of Dementia

Recent research indicates that potentially modifiable socioeconomic and 'lifestyle' factors (e.g. low educational attainment, smoking, physical inactivity, social isolation, etc.) are responsible for about 35 per cent of the risk of developing dementia (Livingston et al., 2017), and the other 65 per cent of the risk is attributed to non-modifiable factors, with ageing being the biggest single factor. But the variety of factors and potentially complex interactions between them mean that it is impossible to say with certainty what caused dementia to develop for any single individual. The evidence, useful for so many purposes, can nevertheless give rise to pejorative or incorrect values-based perceptions of dementia (e.g. dementia is the person's fault for leading an 'unhealthy' lifestyle, dementia is just part of growing old), which can cause friction among carers and practitioners and misrepresentations of dementia in the media. Again, the wheel may squeak because of values being applied to a skewed view of the evidence, but used correctly the evidence is helpful.

Treatment Interventions, Prognosis, and Hope

There is currently no evidence base that clearly points to an intervention(s) which cures or permanently stops the development of any form of dementia (apart from HIV-AIDS dementia, other infective causes of dementia, or normal pressure hydrocephalus if treated in time). For example, various medications, as we've discussed in Chapter 8, may be prescribed for Alzheimer's disease that temporarily improve some symptoms. There is also a range of psychosocial interventions, including formal psychological treatments, such as cognitive stimulation therapy, and more eclectic approaches involving, for example, participatory arts, where there are varying degrees of evidence indicating some benefits for people with dementia.

An evidence base involving a wide range of interventions, all of limited effectiveness, can easily give rise to values, and conflicting values, becoming central in decisions about the care provided to someone with dementia. A person with Alzheimer's disease, their relatives, and health care professionals might all disagree about the use of medication based upon differences in their values and views of drug treatments, causing the wheel to squeak. Yet this should not result in the available evidence about a possible drug treatment being ignored.

Where a prognosis for a progressive, potentially terminal illness is not positive and treatment options are limited, there is the very real risk that the sounds of the squeaky wheel may be dominated by despair and frustration. Facts and evidence may be helpful in these situations, but good communication, honesty, compassion, therapeutic rapport, and understanding the values of the person with dementia and their carers are likely to be equally as important, if not more so. Practitioners should be open to discussing what a person can do to plan ahead, signposting them to different forms of support depending on what they most need, and considering different interventions, even if some have only a very limited evidence base. The importance of interventions that have an evidence base for improving a person's mood and wellbeing should not be underestimated, even if they do not directly affect the person's dementia. Depression, anxiety, and quality of the relationship with a carer are much better predictors of quality of life for a person with dementia than the progress or severity of the actual dementia, so therapeutic and psychosocial interventions that address these issues should be considered (Woods, 2012).

The subjective experience of dementia, choice, and consent

Where dementia affects a person's perception and understanding of the world, their memory, and their ability to communicate, it becomes very difficult for them to participate in discussions about their dementia. It is also very difficult for carers and practitioners fully to know what the person is experiencing and how best to respond. A 'reality' being experienced by a person with dementia that is clearly different from what is actually around them (such as believing a deceased parent or spouse is still alive, a close family member is an imposter, or a care home they are living in is a cruise ship) may be the result of dementia but can also be infused with the person's life story, values, beliefs, and needs. It may be a complete reality for the person. Their values are therefore likely to be very different from that of family members and practitioners around them. Both the values and the 'facts' (as perceived by the person with dementia compared to the perception of others) may be squeaking in these situations!

But as we mentioned in Chapter 6, it may be possible to work with the person's values in these situations in different ways, and there is also some evidence to draw upon about what different realities and beliefs may mean to a person with dementia and how best to respond (Mental Health Foundation, 2015). Even where the wheel is exceptionally squeaky, VBP reminds us that we should still look for what evidence there is, in addition to paying attention to the values that are being expressed.

The effects dementia has on cognition, memory, and communication also pose major difficulties concerning choice and consent. As dementia progresses, a person's ability to express their wishes and preferences, to give or withhold consent, is likely to become increasingly compromised and make decisions about care and treatment more complicated. The squeak in the wheel may become increasingly mysterious as it becomes harder to know what the person's preference would be as new situations and questions arise involving how best to care or support them. While public policy regarding disability rights and social care in many countries (and required by the United Nations Convention on the Rights of Persons with Disabilities) has gone in the direction of promoting a person's right to make choices and have control and independence, this can result in tensions where a person's disability progressively limits their own ability to exercise these functions (Laybourne et al., 2014).

Where dementia places major limitations on communication and cognition, establishing facts or evidence, either individually or collectively, becomes extremely challenging. For many people emotions and memory still seem to play an important role in the way a person understands the world around them, but it's harder to understand how they may still be using facts and values. Establishing what their preference or consent would be involves various processes using both rights-based and evidence-based approaches. These include:

- Adhering to legal frameworks for mental capacity and competency (e.g. supported decision making with advocates, carers, etc.) to identify the person's will and preference (or making best-interests decisions if allowed to do so);
- Encouraging and supporting a person with dementia to record their own life histories, advance plans, statements, directives, refusals of treatment, etc., and/ or authorizing others to make decisions on their behalf if they are unable to do so themselves through powers of attorney. These can cover health, social care, welfare, accommodation, property, and financial decisions, incorporating personal and religious beliefs, and are often recognized by law;
- Exploring different modes of communication. There is evidence to indicate that cognitive impairments or gradual loss of verbal communication does not necessarily mean a person with dementia is unable to express choices. For example, Talking Mats, a simple pictorial way of supporting a person with dementia to express preferences and make decisions, have a good evidence base for people with more severe dementia (Murphy and Oliver, 2013). 'Intensive interaction', an approach adopted from the field of learning disabilities ('adaptive interaction') to communicate with people with dementia who are non-verbal by creating 'conversations' based on behaviours such as sounds, movements, eye contact, and touch, may also provide clues about likes and dislikes (Ellis and Astell, 2017).

One other area of the person's experience of dementia that may create squeaky wheels is where the person is able to research their own condition (e.g. via the Internet) and identifies interventions which they believe will be of benefit. They may identify very relevant interventions, but these may not be available where the person lives, or they may be too costly, or lack sufficient evidence for practitioners to agree to them. There are very few interventions whose efficacy is supported by what is regarded as a robust evidence base (e.g. large randomized controlled trials), yet a large number of psychosocial interventions are supported by evidence which is considered less strong, for example, small qualitative studies (but see Livingston et al., 2014). Providing interventions have not shown to be harmful, practitioners need to be open-minded and supportive of a person with dementia who is keen to play a role in directing their own care. After all, a sense of agency is likely to benefit the person's wellbeing. Certainly, practitioners and carers should be very clear about why they are rejecting an intervention.

Impact of dementia on different groups in society

In this book we have focused mainly on the impact of dementia on individuals, but there is a growing body of evidence indicating differential impacts of the condition on various groups in society. Not all practitioners and dementia services are necessarily aware of this, and it can therefore be the source of several different squeaky wheels. Usually practitioners cannot resolve these at a macro level, but it is important to be aware of them and the relevant evidence in order that appropriate care and support can be provided to an individual, taking into account their particular demographic group. While care and treatment should be tailored to the individual, they also need to be culturally responsive and appropriate for all groups that need them. Here are some examples of demographic factors where dementia can have a differential effect (see also Williamson and McCarthy, 2016):

- Gender (both women and men);
- Age (especially people under the age of 65 with early-onset dementia and the 'very old');
- Black, Asian, and minority ethnic (BAME) communities;
- People with disabilities (in addition to dementia as a disability);
- People who are lesbian, gay, bisexual, trans, + (LGBT+)[1];
- People with different socioeconomic status.

There are a number of ways in which the impact of dementia may interact with other factors leading to differential impacts, including:

- Stereotyped perceptions of who is most likely to experience dementia;
- Differences in life course, life expectancy, or life opportunities affecting risk, prevalence, or ability to use dementia services;
- Limited awareness of dementia, fear or concern about using mainstream providers, or stigma, preventing uptake of services;
- Experience of direct discrimination based upon demographic characteristics such as age, gender, ethnicity, sexual orientation, disability, and so on;
- Communication difficulties and other barriers to accessing or using services experienced by particular groups (potential indirect discrimination).

All of these can create squeaky wheels, on their own or in combination, in the way individuals or groups in society affected by dementia are treated. Increased awareness, knowledge, and understanding of the interrelationship between dementia and demographic factors are important for practitioners working wherever there are diverse populations. Information about dementia, access and design of dementia services, provision of care, and clinical practice should take into account demography and relevant evidence of what works with different groups. But where discrimination, societal changes, or policy

---

[1] '+' refers to other sexual and gender minority groups.

decisions are clear factors in creating differential impacts for the prevalence of dementia, values involving oversight, ignorance, fear, or prejudice are usually involved. Because evidence clearly indicates many of the differential (and deleterious) effects this has on different groups, values *plus* facts creates a squeaky wheel. A consensus has developed in many countries that the effects of this squeaky wheel are unacceptable, and a response has been framed in terms of rights and laws prohibiting discrimination in the way business and public services treat people with certain demographic characteristics. These rights, although based upon values, acquire the apparent solidity of facts by being enshrined in law, universally applicable in any situation they relate to, and immutable unless changed by a country's legislature. Facts and values become blurred, and although rights may help oil one squeaky wheel, they can inadvertently create others.

Carers

Family members and friends of people with dementia who are involved in their care are, as we discussed in Chapter 6, a crucial component of the support that the person receives. It is estimated that in the UK the costs of unpaid care provided by family and friends amounts to £11.6 billion, or 44 per cent of the total cost of dementia (Prince et al., 2014). Yet the effects of dementia on a person's behaviour, emotions, interactions, and even recognition of family members and friends may not only cause them distress but can also be very upsetting for carers, who both wish to care for the person and need advice, support, care, and respite themselves. But we have seen that carers themselves may have diverse views and values. In other words, carers may generate, quite legitimately, their own squeaky wheels.

In many situations providing information, guidance, and support and explaining (on the basis of available evidence) which interventions may work and which probably won't may overcome these difficulties. Not acknowledging the facts of a long-standing, often intimate relationship between the person with dementia and a carer, the values contained in that relationship, and the knowledge the carer has of the person with dementia (together with the person's own knowledge) will only make the wheel squeak more. Where the 'facts' described by the person with dementia are not congruent with the 'facts' described by the carer, practitioners should make particular efforts to establish the facts for themselves. 'Think facts; think values' will involve drawing upon the facts of a person's life, involving family and friends, and being cognizant of the values in play. This approach, along with knowledge of the evidence for possible interventions, will be helpful in determining next steps.

As well as showing the variety of situations where squeaky wheels can be heard, all these examples clearly illustrate the first principle of our Manifesto (*dementia as humanity*). Dementia is so much more than a health condition: it both affects and manifests itself in a person's sense of identity, subjective experience of the world around them, and their relationships. The same is often true for carers. Dementia is also a condition that can have differential impacts on different communities, emphasizing that it is a condition experienced by both individuals and groups in society.

And when one considers in a bit more detail the epidemiology, symptomatology, and treatment of dementia, these reflect the first principle of the Manifesto too. 'Lifestyle' factors modifiable by individuals are often also socioeconomic factors which are modifiable by political systems, ideologies, policies, and corporate and political decisions. Food with high sugar and salt content sell well but are bad for both one's cardiovascular and cognitive systems. Symptoms often reflect a person's life story, relationships, and place in society, and treatments may involve a whole range of social interactions, connections, and people.

What all these areas of dementia care also show is that despite the evidence base being limited, there are still resources that can be used when values are in conflict and the wheel is squeaking. Randomized controlled trials (RCTs) using quantitative methodologies have shown some positive results, as in the case of the cholinesterase inhibitors and memantine discussed in Chapter 8. Treatments that can be based on RCTs are limited. Increasingly, however, psychosocial treatments have also been the subject of good quality quantitative research, which includes RCTs. Livingston et al. (2014), in a systematic review, showed that person-centred care, communication skills training, and adapted dementia care mapping (an observational tool) decreased symptomatic and severe agitation in care homes immediately and for up to six months afterwards. They also showed that activities, music therapy, and sensory interventions could decrease agitation. On the other hand, they found no good evidence that aromatherapy and light therapy were efficacious.

In addition, qualitative research is producing evidence in favour of certain sorts of intervention. Rapaport et al. (2017), for instance, conducted a systematic review to try to understand the elements of psychosocial interventions which are associated with better outcomes for people with dementia in care homes. This included quantitative and qualitative studies. The qualitative data showed that staff valued interventions which focused on getting to know, understand, and connect with the residents living with dementia. Often, quantitative data and qualitative data can come together to support the use of a particular intervention. For instance, in a study of dance in care homes, it was possible to show statistically significant benefits (Guzmán et al., 2016), but this finding was supported by the (qualitative) comments of staff and residents (Guzmán et al., 2017). Indeed, the UK's National Institute for Care and Health Excellence (NICE) will use whatever good quality evidence is available in its guidance, and on this basis will make recommendations about both pharmacological and non-pharmacological treatments. For example, its 2006 guidance on supporting people with dementia and their carers stated the following could be used in addition to mainstream medical, behavioural, and other interventions, if available: aromatherapy, multi-sensory stimulation, therapeutic use of music and/or dancing, animal-assisted therapy, and massage (NICE, 2006).

So, it is clearly the case that evidence can support various types of intervention and evidence might be useful when there are clashes of values (i.e. squeaky wheels). But research can also demonstrate and comment on areas where there might be different values. For instance, Poole et al. (2018), through interviews, have shown that people with dementia and family carers do not always share views on what is key to achieving good end-of-life care and that the views of people with dementia and family carers do not always accord with professional consensus on optimal end-of-life care. Squeaky wheels are everywhere in dementia care, which is a reason why the third principle of our Manifesto is so pertinent (*VBP for dementia plus rights*): VBP is obviously applicable to dementia care as one way to provide a framework for support, care, and treatment to all concerned.

Now 'Think Values; Think Facts' – and Think Diagnosis?

To explore the 'squeaky wheel' principle further, let's look at an example that focuses on one key area of dementia care, because it is so fundamental to practice as well as to the subjective experience of dementia, and because it highlights the link between values and facts.

For any health condition, diagnosis is absolutely fundamental. Without a diagnosis, the person experiencing the condition and their family and friends will not know for certain what the problem is, its prognosis, or how it will affect their lives, and they may be unable to make plans for the future. Despite 'a surprising lack of research' looking at the timing of a diagnosis of dementia, 'informed and expert opinion' is generally of the view that an early diagnosis can lead to better outcomes by slowing and stabilizing cognitive and functional decline, treating depression, improving caregiver mood, and delaying moves into residential care (Prince et al., 2011). A diagnosis of dementia as a progressive and terminal condition, with its associated cognitive, physical, mental, and communication impairments, should also provide access to the following (though not necessarily by right or without a financial charge):

- Specialist health treatments, psychosocial interventions, and other services;
- Social care services;
- Specialist accommodation, residential, and nursing care;
- Disability benefits and services;
- Protection from discrimination under disability legislation.

If one dares say it, *the fact is* that without a dementia diagnosis, people do not have rights to a whole range of services and protections. (It's interesting to note here how 'rights' become gateways that allow access to services, even though the gateway may be based upon a whole a range of social, political, and economic values.) They are also unlikely to benefit from evidence-based interventions. The wheel will almost certainly squeak louder as the dementia becomes more severe. To quote the well-known author, Terry Pratchett OBE, who died in in 2015 eight years after being diagnosed with a form of Alzheimer's disease (posterior cortical atrophy), talking about dementia,

> It's a fact, well enshrined in folklore, that if we are to kill the demon then first we have to say its name.
>
> (Williamson, 2008: x)

Pratchett is quoted from a report based on a qualitative study about people's experience of being diagnosed with dementia. Although some people with dementia in the same report described a sense of shock and distress about receiving a diagnosis, others were relieved:

> I was relieved really that what I had been trying to convince people had been verified.
>
> (person with dementia in Williamson, 2008: 28)

> My initial reaction was disappointment because I had been hoping it was something else. But both of us, it is very interesting really, both of us felt liberated by it.
>
> (family carer in Williamson, 2008: 28)

These sentiments echo the views of people with dementia from another earlier qualitative study:

> I would shoot the person that tried to keep it [a dementia diagnosis] back from me. I really think it's an absolute disgrace, you should be told at the earliest moment, even if people say to you it might be that, we'll have to test if, even tell them then. Then if you want to ignore it, ignore it if you wish, but it's your choice, it's not the doctor's choice, or the carer's choice, it's your choice, and you should be given that choice.
>
> (Pratt and Wilkinson, 2001)

Yet in 2011, Alzheimer Disease International estimated that as many as 28 million of the world's 36 million people with dementia had yet to receive a diagnosis and therefore did not have access to treatment, information, and care (Prince et al., 2011). In 2014, it was estimated that around half of the people living with dementia in Europe had never been diagnosed (Alzheimer Europe, 2014). Taking England as an example, in 2007 it was estimated that only one-third of people with dementia received a formal diagnosis at any time in their illness (National Audit Office, 2007). According to the UK government's Department of Health, this figure had risen, on average, to two-thirds of people affected by dementia in 2016, although there were considerable regional variations (Department of Health, 2016).

So, despite the fact that there may well be concrete benefits from getting a dementia diagnosis, the wheel squeaks for many individuals (and services) where a diagnosis is not available. A number of reasons are associated with why some people don't get a diagnosis of dementia, based on both values and facts. These include:

Stigma

Dementia still carries a stigma based upon values associated with fear, ignorance, and prejudice. People may avoid seeking a diagnosis (or finding out what the problem is) when they first experience its effects. Although we should all agree that there should not be stigma associated with dementia, there is plenty of evidence to show that this stigma exists in the way it is presented by the media, in people's experience of discrimination, and so on. In this sense, unfortunately, stigma has an evidence base (Bamford et al., 2014).

People Avoiding a Diagnosis

For several different reasons, some people do not go and see a doctor when they first experience the effects of dementia. They may attribute increasing loss of memory, for example, to a natural part of the ageing process. They may not want to find out because of fear. They may just not like going to see a doctor. Again, there are values implicit in not seeking a diagnosis, sometimes based partly on evidence (e.g. that treatment options are limited and only modestly effective). It is also true that, although not an inevitable part of ageing, getting old does increase the risk of developing dementia. It's worth noting that avoiding a diagnosis is a generic health problem: almost half the number of people with cancer in the UK are diagnosed late, which greatly reduces their chances of survival, despite there being much more effective cancer treatment available, particularly if diagnosed early (Incisive Health/Cancer Research UK, 2014).

'Therapeutic Nihilism'

This is the belief that treatment is not possible. Although much less common these days, some doctors and health care professionals avoid diagnosing or telling the person their diagnosis because the treatments available are limited. In the age of austerity politics, they may also be aware (or believe) that services providing care and support for people with dementia are very limited. Doctors may not want to cause the person distress or may say 'it's just part of getting old'. Hence, values, but some facts as well, conspire so that people do not get a diagnosis.

We also need to remember, as discussed in Chapter 8, that the process of diagnosing dementia is often complicated and sometimes imprecise. Evaluative judgements are often made about whether or not someone has dementia. Differentiating between, for example, mild cognitive impairments and early Alzheimer's disease is far from easy. The 'facts' of a score on the Mini-Mental State Examination (MMSE) may indicate that something is wrong, but this needs to be tested over time, perhaps, and other evidence drawn upon, such as the views of carers.

So if someone with the symptoms of dementia goes through a diagnostic process, it neither automatically means they get a diagnosis, nor that the diagnosis is based on irrefutable facts. Furthermore, a doctor may decide not to disclose a diagnosis of dementia to the person but may, or may not, tell a close relative. And even if a person with dementia is given a diagnosis, they may deny it or may choose not to tell anyone, perhaps using the term 'memory problems' instead, for some of the reasons described earlier. The 'fact' of having dementia does not mean that values (and other facts) don't still guide a person's actions or prevent the wheel from squeaking. Let's consider this example.

Vignette - Marta

Marta is 67 and lives by herself in a flat in a large city. She grew up in Spain but came to the UK over 45 years ago to work as a nurse. Her husband died six years ago, and she has two grown-up sons, Marc and Sergio, and a grown-up daughter, Paula. Marc lives and works abroad, but Sergio and Paula live near Marta. Sergio has a family of his own. But Paula, who is the youngest sibling, is single. Marta has one sibling still alive, a brother who lives in Spain. Paula visits her mother regularly, although Sergio only calls in occasionally. Four years ago, Marta started saying that neighbours had been coming into her flat and stealing things although there was no evidence of this and several things she claimed had been stolen were found elsewhere in her flat. She also started phoning all her children in the middle of the night accusing them of never visiting her, yet she had no recollection of making the calls when asked about it the next day.

Although Marta didn't see these incidents as possible problems with her health, she agreed to go with Paula to see the family doctor (GP) because of the anxiety and worry they were causing her. The doctor said that there was nothing to worry about and these kinds of situations were common as one grew older. However, he did refer her to a specialist for some memory tests. Marta went for the tests and the GP informed her that she had mild memory problems but that this was common in old age. However, he then spoke to Paula in private and said that the tests indicated that Marta almost certainly had Alzheimer's disease, but because the prognosis for dementia was so poor and there was no effective treatment, he did not want to worry Marta unduly by telling her. He advised Paula that her mother should have as much social contact as possible, both at home and outside the home, such as continuing to go to her local church.

When Paula told Marc and Sergio what the doctor had said, they were both adamant that their mother should not be told about the Alzheimer's disease. Paula disagreed and argued that their mother had a right to know and that it would make getting help and support easier. Marc became angry. He said Marta shouldn't go to church because it would bring shame on their family. He said it was probably brought on by their mother worrying that Paula was still single and should have had a family by now, so it was her responsibility to look after their mother. He then slammed down the phone. Sergio eventually just shrugged his shoulders and said Paula could try and tell Marta, but she would have to deal with the consequences. The next day Paula spoke with her mother who listened but then became angry and said, 'Are you trying to tell me I'm sick? I think you just want to lock me up somewhere! I'm fine, the doctor said so, he wouldn't lie!'

Paula became Marta's main form of support, which Paula found increasingly stressful. Over the next 18 months Marta's condition deteriorated: she stopped going to church because she thought the priest was 'spying' on her and became increasingly abusive towards her neighbours, whom she accused of being 'out to get me'. When Paula tried to suggest that Marta was imagining these things, Marta got angry with her and accused her of being on their side. When Paula did not challenge Marta, she found herself having to go along with what her mother said, which made her feel very uncomfortable and did little to allay Marta's suspicion and paranoia. If she tried to change the subject or distract her mother, Marta became very suspicious and said that Paula was behaving oddly.

As the dementia progressed, Marta's paranoia increased and she frequently refused or was unable to communicate in English or Spanish, often speaking in Basque instead, the area of Spain where she originally came from. Paula and Sergio both had only limited knowledge of Basque. Marta's self-care deteriorated, but she was insistent that she stayed living in her flat, that she was okay 'because the doctor said so', and kept on saying the word 'fascist'. She refused to go and see the GP, and when he visited her at home at Paula's request, Marta said she was very well and that he could go away. Paula was at a loss what to do. Although Paula continued to visit, at times her mother became angry and told her to go away, saying, 'You are not my daughter, my daughter would never treat me like this, how can I trust you', and also started calling Paula 'Celia', the name of a deceased sister of Marta's.

The situation came to a head when Marta's brother visited, staying at Sergio's house. Marta had a fall coming out of her flat and hit her head on the pavement. A neighbour called an ambulance. Marta resisted going in the ambulance, hitting the paramedics, and shouting, 'Don't lock me up'. She was so resistant that despite a bleeding head wound the police had to be called to escort her in the ambulance to hospital. When she came into the accident and emergency (A&E) department she remained very agitated and was referred for a psychiatric assessment. One of the nurses who was with Marta asked what she did and Marta said she was a nurse. The psychiatrist who came to see her knew a bit of Spanish and said in response, 'You should know all about how a hospital works'. This seemed to calm her down a lot and she started talking about the hospital 'duties' she had. The psychiatrist decided to detain her under the Mental Health Act, because although happy to be in hospital, Marta said she was not a patient and intended to leave soon, despite her head injury (which had been treated but was thought to be serious).

Once in hospital Marta seemed much calmer. She liked following the staff around and offering her help. Marta's key nurse had recently been on both life story training (Gridley et al., 2015) and validation therapy training (Neal and Barton Wright, 2003), and both she and Marta's psychiatrist were familiar with the concept of 'time-shifting', where a person with dementia appears to believe they are at a different time in their life. They asked to speak with Marta's family and through Marta's brother established that Marta left Spain because she had sympathies with the communists and no longer felt safe living there under the fascist president, General Franco. Her deceased sister Celia had disapproved of her politics but did not report her to the authorities. Marta's behaviour was probably because the effect of the dementia was making her believe she was back in Spain, that Paula was Celia, whom she did not trust, and that the priest and her neighbours were fascist sympathizers from the area where she lived.

Marta remained settled on the ward, and discussions began about her discharge from hospital. It was agreed by the family and staff that Marta lacked capacity to decide where to live and, in a best-interests meeting, it was decided that she should move into a care home. The move went remarkably smoothly, partly because the nurse advised the family that they describe the care home as being similar to a nurses' home where Marta had first lived when she came to the UK. Initially they were concerned about lying to their mother, but discussed this and decided that Marta's wellbeing was the priority. Marta liked this idea; she was a bit surprised by the age of the other residents when she moved in, but staff gave her 'nursing jobs' to do in the home (e.g. carrying things for them, helping make teas and coffees), which enabled her to settle in and feel valued. The whole of the family felt relieved and reassured that she was finally getting the care and support she needed. Staff in the home were well trained in best practice dementia care, and Paula in particular liked the home's person-centred values. Although Marta still didn't recognize Paula as her daughter, she no longer associated her in a negative way with Celia and at times thought Paula was 'someone nice' coming to visit her. Although this felt strange to Paula, it meant that she could visit Marta in the home, and even when she thought Paula was Celia she appeared to be relaxed in her company.

Commentary

Marta's story is a story of several squeaky wheels, where there are problems involving values but also facts. We have discussed the reasons why the GP decided not to tell Marta her diagnosis, but it misled her and made it difficult for her to understand what was happening when she was already cognitively impaired, thus making it virtually impossible to provide any helpful interventions and causing a rift within the family (although the GP did not know this would happen).

Of course, gently telling Marta that all the signs indicated that she had Alzheimer's disease might still have resulted in her denying it and believing that the GP was against her. She might have got upset or depressed. But in terms of facts and evidence, Marta denying that she had dementia does not appear any worse than her not being told at all. And if she had become upset or depressed, the support of her family and interventions for depression could have alleviated this. There is no evidence that we know of that shows better outcomes for people if they are not told their diagnosis, deny it, or do not disclose it. There is some evidence both that objective outcomes and the subjective experience of the person with dementia and their carers are better if people are diagnosed and diagnosed early. The evidence is thin, meaning it is scanty and not always top-class, but if a variety of interventions might alleviate distress and increase wellbeing, in the absence of harmful effects, it is easy to argue it is worth pursuing. These decisions should be based upon VBP's balanced decision-making approach, involving all parties.

Telling (or Not Telling) the Truth (Again)

In terms of values and rights, didn't Marta have a right to be told the truth that she probably had Alzheimer's? The GP was also perhaps reluctant to tell her because it wasn't a definitive diagnosis. But surely professionals need to be able to communicate uncertainties and probabilities as well? Williamson and Kirtley (2016) recognized that avoiding causing distress and ensuring wellbeing may at times mean that one has to 'go along with' what the person with dementia is believing, but this should only occur when there is evidence that truth-telling consistently causes harm or distress. Truth-telling, certainly as a starting point, is an important moral value for most people, and is also crucial in terms of someone being able to exercise their rights fully, based upon respect for autonomy. Marta's decision-making ability was compromised partly by the effects of her dementia but also, arguably, by her not being told her diagnosis. Finally, Marta might not have chosen to receive additional support from specialist dementia services or third-sector organisations, but at least she would have had the choice.

We have given the story a positive ending. It doesn't always work out like this. But the happy ending came out of another squeaky wheel, a very difficult hospital admission. Again, values were a clear problem – autonomy versus protection: Marta's resistance to being in hospital versus the professional belief that she needed to be admitted. The situation involved facts, but these were being interpreted differently according to different sets of values. Marta's were based upon a very different understanding of what was happening to her from those around her. Using an evidence base from life story work, validation therapy, and an understanding of 'time shifting', the nurse and the psychiatrist, in partnership with Marta's family, were able to understand what lay behind her behaviour. Her suspicion and paranoia indicated a psychotic component to her dementia. It could have been treated with medication in the form of antipsychotics to sedate her, and there is evidence to support this, along with evidence of the potential harms of antipsychotics (Ballard and Howard, 2006). In any event, the professionals used a different approach, which also worked, and engaged more sensitively with the different reality that Marta was experiencing. However, it required a values-based decision that truth-telling was not the most important part of their response. They chose to go along with Marta's reality by acting as if she was still a nurse in order to reassure her and enable her to have a sense of wellbeing. The family and the care home also agreed to act in this way – they had the cognitive capacity to do this, whereas Marta's dementia prevented her from understanding that she was no longer a nurse. They could adapt; Marta couldn't. Marta's hospital admission involved detaining her under the law. The resistance that many people with dementia exhibit when compulsorily detained is in one way a clear illustration of a clash of values creating a squeaky wheel: autonomy versus protection. But although laws are based upon values, they also have the feel of being facts; they usually involve a clear right and wrong, and laws cannot easily be changed. By having an awareness and understanding of the law and rights more generally, squeaky wheels caused by this blurring of facts and values can be averted.

Rights

The third principle of our Manifesto states: 'Using VBP in partnership with evidence-based practice *and an applied understanding of rights* will significantly enhance both the quality of life and the quality of care for people living with dementia' (emphasis added).

So far in this chapter we have talked about the squeaky wheel in relation to values and facts. We have suggested that by 'thinking values, thinking facts' the wheel may turn smoothly again, as if the 'unified, two fields' view of facts and values (see Figure 1.2) had been achieved and the circle (squeaky wheel) was fixed. But values can sometimes be a bit more like the 'petal' image in Figure 1.1, showing the wide range of sources from where values can come. In other words, even if the Fact + Value model is aligned (as in Figure 1.2), there may still be jarring caused by different values coming into conflict with each other. Of course, this (and how to deal with it) is partly what this book is all about. But it is also worth remembering the particular challenges, described in Chapter 2, where dementia can cause additional disagreements about values, but particularly about the issue of rights.

Let's go back to Marta. Although Marta seems settled in the home, she quite often tries to leave, saying she has to go to work. When there are enough staff available someone often walks out with Marta 'to go to work with her'. Marta quite quickly forgets where she is going and is happy to return to the home. Sometimes, however, Marta is prevented from leaving the home. The manager of the home realizes that because Marta lacks mental capacity to consent to being in the home, even though mostly she is quite settled there, she is almost certainly being deprived of her liberty, which is a breach of her human rights (Article 5 of the European Convention on Human Rights, as applied by the UK's Human Rights Act 1998) unless authorized by law. According to current law in England and Wales, Marta must therefore be assessed and should probably come under the Deprivation of Liberty Safeguards (DoLS), a part of the MCA.

However, when the manager discusses making a referral for Marta to be assessed under DoLS with staff and Marta's family, they become frustrated and upset. Some staff, and Paula in particular, believe the assessment process will confuse or upset her and make her think she isn't safe there. Paula says that 'those DoLS things make the home sound like a prison'.

This example shows how values and facts may appear to be aligned and both staff and family are in agreement, but there can still be squeaky wheels. With DoLS, the squeaky wheel is that Marta's human rights are seen to represent a problem rather than a protection.

There are possible ways around these difficulties. Marta needs to be consistently reassured that she's safely back at home with the other 'nurses'. Ensuring that the assessment for DoLS is done swiftly, and if possible by practitioners whom Marta knows, may minimize any confusion it causes her. Because other residents are under DoLS, it could be described to Marta as a way of making sure all the 'nurses' living in the home are safe (as well as explaining to Marta's family exactly what DoLS are).

The real purpose of the example is to remind us that values come in all sorts of shapes and sizes. Values contained in laws such as mental capacity legislation must be respected and made to work in as beneficial a way as possible for the person with the disability or illness (and often equally, their carers). When rights are expressed in legal frameworks (as opposed to rhetorical expressions of 'rights' without legal substantiation), they also contain a factual quality; if a DoLS assessment is not carried out, it could be a violation of Marta's human rights and the law (whatever one's views about this) is being broken. Rights therefore have a quality of being a coin with two sides: an expression of values but also the seeming immutability of facts when expressed in legal frameworks. So VBP provides a good process to work in partnership with a rights-based approach and, also, situations may necessitate such an approach. To some extent the same duality can also be said of values contained in professional codes of conduct, organizational policies, and procedures which should be service-user focused, where violations can have serious consequences – but rights illustrate the point well because they are universal and more socially embedded. This discussion also calls to mind our second Manifesto principle: there are the facts of dementia as a disease, but the implications of *dementia as a disability* are mostly realized in terms of rights, with correlative duties for those who should support and care for people who live with dementia.

The example also reminds us that there can be a blurring between values and moral 'rights' – think of truth telling – such that rights, whilst being considered, may perhaps be compromised in relation to the wellbeing of the person.[2] Furthermore, although truth-telling can be seen as a moral right, not causing unnecessary distress could also be called

---

[2] It's important to note that Article 25(1) of the United Nations Declaration on Human Rights states that '[e]veryone has the right to a standard of living adequate for the health and *wellbeing* of himself [sic] and of his family' (emphasis added). In England, the Care Act 2015 places wellbeing as its central principle for the provision of services to people with care and support needs. In this sense, the right to wellbeing has legal status.

a moral right and indeed a human right: Article 3 of the European Convention on Human Rights states that '[n]o-one shall be subjected to torture or to inhuman or degrading treatment or punishment'. Could persistence in telling the truth to a person with dementia which causes them distress be considered 'inhuman treatment'?

We are not advocating that all professionals have to be experts in law. But they do need to be mindful of rights as well as values and facts. And professionals should not be frightened of the law. Wellbeing is an important and useful concept. And as we shall see in Chapter 12, although there are criticisms of legal frameworks for substitute decision making, such as best interests (because they are not compliant with the United Nations Convention on the Rights of Persons with Disabilities), the frameworks do provide helpful processes for making decisions about care and treatment. A rights-based approach is not just a requirement when it involves the law, it can work in partnership with VBP. And VBP emphasizes how crucial it is to establish what values, facts, and rights are in play for the person with dementia, carers, and professionals when the wheel squeaks.

Key Points

- In some respects, dementia in its totality is a squeaky wheel – thinking of it in these terms is not to make it problematic, but to highlight the complicated interrelationships involving people, facts, and values. But squeaky wheels are ubiquitous in human life in general, irrespective of dementia. Everyday disagreements involve squeaky wheels.
- But there can be particularly squeaky wheels in dementia care. These can arise from difficulties and disagreements in the care of an individual with dementia and may involve family members and friends who do not understand what is happening or are distressed. They can also arise from the needs of particular population groups affected by dementia. And they reflect how dementia is a touchstone for understanding a person's place in the world.
- Because our knowledge of dementia and how to treat or respond appropriately to someone with dementia (especially as it becomes more severe) is limited, facts and values become entangled. What people believe about dementia – their values – can often feel like reality or solid evidence, and using evidence often requires judgements based on values. Being open about this complexity and uncertainty and enabling as much as possible a person with dementia and carers to understand this are fundamental in how VBP is applied.
- Squeaky wheels require open discussion about values but also consideration of evidence. Evidence may be limited, conflicting, and involve several options. There may be no RCTs to draw upon, but there may be qualitative evidence about what can work. We should be prepared to consider and use more eclectic evidence or evidence that might challenge one's assumptions. Values come back into play when making decisions involving a diverse range of approaches based on limited evidence.
- Rights also add to the gritty mix of facts and values that cause the wheel to squeak. They contain elements of facts and values, but when enshrined in legal frameworks they should not be ignored – and may even help in the same way that viewing dementia as a disability also helps.
- So, when squeaky wheels occur – 'Think values; think facts; but think rights too!'

References

Aalten, P., Verhey, F. R., Boziki, M., et al. (2007). Neuropsychiatric syndromes in dementia: Results from the European Alzheimer disease consortium. *Dementia and Geriatric Cognitive Disorders* 24, 457–63.

Alzheimer Europe. (2014). *Dementia in Europe Yearbook 2014. National Care Pathways for People with Dementia Living at Home.* Luxembourg: Alzheimer Europe. Available via: www.alzheimer-europe .org/Publications/Dementia-in-Europe-Yearbooks (last accessed 30 December 2017).

Ballard, C., and Howard, R. (2006). Neuroleptic drugs in dementia: Benefits and harm. *Nature Reviews Neuroscience*, 7, 492–500.

Bamford, S.-M., Holley-Moore, G., and Jessica Watson, J., eds. (2014). *A Compendium of Essays: New Perspectives and Approaches to Understanding Dementia and Stigma.* London: The International Longevity Centre-UK. Available via: www.ilcuk.org .uk/index.php/publications (last accessed 30 December 2017).

Corey-Bloom, J., and Rafii, M. S. (2017). The natural history of Alzheimer's disease. In D. Ames, J. O'Brien, and A. Burns, eds., *Dementia*, 5th edn. Boca Raton, London, and New York: CRC Press, Taylor & Francis Group, pp. 453–69.

Department of Health. (2009). *Living Well with Dementia: A National Dementia Strategy.* London: Department of Health. Access via: www.gov.uk/government/ publications/living-well-with-dementia-a-national-dementia-strategy (last accessed 30 December 2017).

(2016). *Prime Minister's Challenge on Dementia 2020; Implementation Plan.* London: Department of Health. Available via: www.gov.uk/government/ publications/challenge-on-dementia-2020-implementation-plan (last accessed 30 December 2017).

Ellis, M., and Astell, A. (2017). *Adaptive Interaction and Dementia: How to Communicate without Speech.* London: Jessica Kingsley Publishers.

Fratiglioni, L., De Ronchi, D., and Aguera-Torres, H. (1999). Worldwide prevalence and incidence of dementia. *Drugs and Aging* 15, 365–75.

Gridley, K., Brooks, J., Birks, Y., et al. (2015). *Life Story Work in Dementia Care.* North Yorkshire: University of York, Social Policy Research Unit. Available via: www.york.ac.uk/inst/spru/research/ pdf/LifeStorySum.pdf (last accessed 30 December 2017).

Guzmán, A., Freeston, M., Rochester, L., Hughes, J. C., and James, I. A. (2016). Psychomotor Dance Therapy Intervention (DANCIN) for people with dementia in care homes: A multiple-baseline single-case study. *International Psychogeriatrics*, 28(10): 1695–715. http://dx.doi.org/ 10.1017/S104161021600051X

Guzmán, A., Robinson, L., Rochester, L, James, I. A., and Hughes, J. C. (2017). A process evaluation of a Psychomotor Dance Therapy Intervention (DANCIN) for behaviour change in dementia: Attitudes and beliefs of participating residents and staff. *International Psychogeriatrics*, 29(2): 313–22. http://dx.doi.org/10.1017/ S104161021600171X

Incisive Health/Cancer Research UK. (2014). *Saving Lives, Averting Costs.* London: Cancer Research UK. Available via: www .cancerresearchuk.org/sites/default/files/ saving_lives_averting_costs.pdf (last accessed 30 December2017).

Laybourne, A., Jepson, M., Williamson, T., et al. (2014). Beginning to explore the experience of managing a direct payment for someone with dementia: The perspective of suitable people and adult social care practitioners. *Dementia* 15, 125–40.

Livingston, G., Sommerlad, A., Orgeta, V., et al. (2017). Dementia prevention, intervention, and care. *The Lancet*, 390, 2673–734.

Livingston, G., Kelly, L., Lewis-Holmes, E., et al. (2014). Non-pharmacological interventions for agitation in dementia: Systematic review of randomised controlled trials. *British Journal of Psychiatry*, 205, 436–42.

McKeith, I. G. (2017). Dementia with Lewy bodies: A clinical overview. In D. Ames, J.

O'Brien and A. Burns, eds., *Dementia,* 5th edn. Boca Raton, London, and New York: CRC Press, Taylor & Francis Group, pp. 703–13.

McKeith, I. G., Dickson, D. W., Lowe, J., et al. (2005). Diagnosis and management of dementia with Lewy bodies. Third report of the DLB consortium. *Neurology* **65,** 1863–72.

Mental Health Foundation. (2015). *Dementia-What Is Truth? Exploring the Real Experience of People Living with More Severe Dementia. A Mental Health Foundation National Inquiry. A Rapid Literature Review.* London: Mental Health Foundation. www.mentalhealth .org.uk/sites/default/files/Dementia per cent20truth per cent20inquiry per cent20lit per cent20review per cent20FINAL per cent20(3).pdf (last accessed 27 September 2018).

Murphy, J., and Oliver, T. M. (2013). The use of Talking Mats to support people with dementia and their carers to make decisions together. *Health and Social Care in the Community* **21,** 171–80.

National Audit Office. (2007). *Improving Services and Support for People with Dementia.* London: The Stationery Office). www.nao .org.uk/report/improving-services-and-support-for-people-with-dementia/ (last accessed 27 September 2018).

Neal, M., and Barton Wright, P. (2003). Validation therapy for dementia. *Cochrane Database of Systematic Reviews,* Issue 3. Art. No.: CD001394. doi: 10.1002/14651858.CD001394

NICE. (2006). *Dementia: Supporting People with Dementia and Their Carers in Health and Social Care. [Clinical Guidelines 42].* London: National Institute for Health and Care Excellence. Available via: www.nice .org.uk/Guidance/CG42 (last accessed 30 December 2017).

Poole, M., McLellan, E., Bamford, C., et al. (2018). End of life care: A qualitative study comparing the views of people with dementia and family carers. *Palliative Medicine* **32**(3), 631–642. http://dx.doi .org/10.1177/026921631776033.

Pratt, R., and Wilkinson, H. (2001). *Tell Me the Truth.* London: Mental Health Foundation.

Available via: www.mentalhealth.org.uk/ publications/tell-me-truth (last accessed 30 December 2017).

Prince, M., Bryce, R., and Ferri, C. (2011). *Alzheimer's Disease International World Alzheimer Report 2011: The Benefits of Early Diagnosis and Intervention.* London: Alzheimer's Disease International. Available via: www.alz.co.uk/research/world-report-2011 (accessed 30 December 2017).

Prince, M., Knapp, M., Guerchet., M, et al. (2014). *Dementia UK Update.* London: Alzheimer's Society. Available via: http:// eprints.lse.ac.uk/59437/1/Dementia_UK_ Second_edition_-_Overview.pdf (accessed 30 December 2017).

Rapaport, P., Livingston, G., Murray, J., Mulla, A., and Cooper, C. (2017). Systematic review of the effective components of psychosocial interventions delivered by care home staff to people with dementia. *BMJ Open* **7,** e014177. doi:10.1136/ bmjopen-2016-014177

Williamson, T. (2008). *Dementia: Out of the Shadows.* London: Alzheimer's Society. Available via: www.mentalhealth.org.uk/ sites/default/files/out_of_the_shadows.pdf (accessed 6 June 2018).

Williamson, T., and Kirtley, A. (2016). *What Is Truth? An Inquiry About Truth, Lying, Different Realities and Beliefs in Dementia Care (Review of Evidence and Report).* London: Mental Health Foundation. Available via: www.mentalhealth.org.uk/ publications/what-truth-inquiry-about-truth-and-lying-dementia-care (accessed 26 December 2017).

Williamson, T., and McCarthy, R. (2016). *Dementia: Equity and Rights.* London: Health & Care Voluntary Sector Strategic Partner Programme. Available at: https:// nationallgbtpartnershipdotorg.files .wordpress.com/2016/04/2016-dementia-equity-and-rights.pdf (accessed 30 December 2017).

Woods, B. (2012). Well-being and dementia: How can it be achieved? *Quality in Ageing and Older Adults,* **13**(3), 205–11.

Zekry, D., Hauw, J.-J., and Gold, G. (2002). Mixed dementia: Epidemiology, diagnosis, and treatment. *Journal of the American Geriatric Society* **50,** 1431–38.

Communication, End of Life, and Values

Topics covered in this chapter
- This chapter is about communication, including elements of good communication and its importance.
- We suggest that palliative care, good quality, person-centred dementia care, and VBP all share important components, one of which is the need for good communication.
- We also discuss advance care plans, the use of antibiotics, eating and drinking (including PEG feeding), and resuscitation, which are all topics that crop up in connection with palliative care in dementia.
- The connections between VBP and palliative dementia care are also apparent in the European Association's White Paper on palliative care for people with dementia.
- All of this links with the three principles of our Manifesto: *dementia as humanity, dementia as disease and disability, and VBP for dementia plus rights*.

Take-away message for practice
Dementia requires good communication, but this is especially so at the end of life. It is also required as part and parcel of good dementia care, good palliative care, and good VBP.

Dementia as a Disease of Communication

We all know how important language is in everyday life. It may seem odd to suggest, but dementia can be regarded as a disorder of language. We naturally think of dementia as a disorder of memory. This is encouraged, perhaps, by the scientific paradigm which emphasized memory deficits partly because they were easy to measure. But, first, it is not just a condition that affects memory. The definition of dementia stresses that it is a global cognitive disorder, which means that it will affect more than just one cognitive domain, such as memory. In fact, often problems with communication are much more frustrating for the person living with dementia than problems with memory. Second, there are types of dementia which mainly affect language. One example is semantic dementia, which causes problems with the meaning of words. There is also a type of dementia called logopenic primary progressive aphasia, which is thought to be a variety of Alzheimer's disease that affects the person's ability to name and to repeat things. Third, even if dementia only affected memory, not being able to remember something does affect communication.

It means we cannot recall the names of people, we cannot remember what has been said, we cannot remember what has recently happened. And all of this would affect our ability to engage in lucid conversation. Finally, and unfortunately, as dementia progresses it always affects language, and eventually most people living with advanced dementia develop aphasia; that is, they cannot speak.

Much work has been done on communication for people living with dementia (Allan and Killick, 2010). Of course, there are two aspects to communication. There is both output and input. Output involves speaking, but will also include gestures, expressions, and other non-verbal manifestations. Input means understanding, but this involves both the central workings of the brain and the ability to hear and see. Although it is difficult, it is possible to help people with communication difficulties. Fixing things that can be fixed – for instance, by improving hearing and vision – will be helpful. Our responses to people with dementia will also be key. We can be supportive, give time, reduce anxiety, listen attentively so that we can grasp the person's meaning, and help them in a sensitive manner.

In Steven Sabat's seminal work, *The Experience of Alzheimer's Disease: Life Through a Tangled Veil*, we are presented with numerous examples of how important communication is to people living with dementia. Dr M is a 75-year-old woman who had always been highly competent and intelligent and had enjoyed 'a life-long love affair with words' (Sabat, 2001: 62). Consider, then, this exchange with Professor Sabat:

DR M: My talking is very much worse. Really wo, wo, very wo, um hum.

SRS: Really – you do think it's worse.

DR M: Oh ya, maybe you will tell me otherwise.

SRS: What makes you think it's worse?

DR M: Um, it, ta, ta, becau, the, I was in another area and uh, the connection with people was different as with here...

...

DR M: My connection with people was, was not there. And that's, I think that, I think I should say this very much uh, I can't speak as well – that's the thing is.

SRS: Um hum.

DR M: And apparently, since I was a child uh, I was a good talker. And that is and also I, that's because that, and now it's different because among the may [many] important things, I can't talk to people. (Sabat, 2001: 74–75)

We can sense here how the language problem is threatening to undermine her sense of herself as a person worthy of respect. We give her back her sense of self-respect by our attitude to her as a person, which, by the by – as Sabat demonstrates so movingly at times – is also the way we encourage her communication. By taking time with her, by helping her (a process Sabat calls 'repair') and not undermining her, we allow her to continue to communicate as best she can. We show that she is valued and that what she values is valued, and these things are intrinsic to her standing as a person.

Other approaches have also been found useful. 'Talking Mats' have been developed to aid communication (Murphy and Oliver, 2013). Picture cards are used, which the person living with dementia can arrange and rearrange, for example, to indicate things which might be important to him or her. Intensive or adaptive interaction is an approach which has been found helpful in advanced dementia (Ellis and Astell, 2017). It involves getting to know the person and his or her ways of communicating despite any impairments. Our aim in this chapter, however, is not to provide an overview of issues to do with communication in dementia (for which the reader might wish to consult Killick and Allan, 2001), but to consider how VBP is relevant to communication in the advanced stages of dementia when normal communication has been lost.

Case Scenario - Mr Youakim (1)

Mr Youakim was diagnosed with mixed Alzheimer's and vascular dementia when he was 74 years old. He is now 86 years old. When he was 81 he was admitted to a care home. His wife had died that year and, without her support, it became difficult to help Mr Youakim to remain in the community. He still has a supportive family, who visit frequently. A daughter lives near the care home and visits every day. Another daughter lives abroad but visits twice a year and rings the home once a month. There is a son, too, who lives at the other end of the country and visits about every two months. After his admission, for about a year, Mr Youakim was quite agitated. It was recognized that he was probably grieving for his wife and was certainly upset to find himself in a care home. His dementia was advanced by this time, and with his speech now poor, it was not even clear that he was always able to recall that his wife had died.

Despite the staff trying to understand what he needed, they had to resort to a variety of drugs to try to control his agitation. He suffered some falls, perhaps as a result of the medication. Gradually, however, Mr Youakim settled. He became more sedentary. For about a year, although not mobile, it was still possible to elicit simple 'yes' and 'no' answers to direct questions. Staff who knew him well could tell when he was distressed and agitated and when he was not. Occasionally he would show humour, smiling or laughing at jokes made by staff. But at other times he would be disgruntled. He developed a series of chest infections, after which he was much frailer. It was difficult for him to sit up straight, and a decision was made to nurse him in bed. At about this time Mr Youakim lost the ability to speak completely. Staff still felt that he understood what they were saying to him, but this became less certain. He is now totally dependent for all of his day-to-day needs, including washing, eating, and going to the toilet.

Communication: Being a Person

Language, it is often said, marks us out as human beings. Loss of language can undermine our standing as human persons. Nevertheless, communication is not solely dependent on spoken language. The reason communication is so basic is that it is part of the way in which we are situated with others. It is this situating context that positions us as human beings. We can be placed in what Sabat calls 'malignant positioning' (Sabat, 2001: 124–25) as other, as deficient, as incapable, and so forth, which is particularly so if our language is problematic. Being a person involves communication because we, as persons, are quintessentially social, interconnected in part by language. But in the absence of language, to the extent that we can still convey meaning by whatever means, we can still communicate. If, however, communication depends (as it does) on those around us interacting with us, then to some extent it can be said that my communicative abilities are in part maintained by the communicative efforts made by others. In short, my standing as a person is maintained by others and chiefly by the many and varied ways in which they communicate with me.

In the case of someone like Mr Youakim, the importance of gestures becomes obvious. In addition, the importance of others is equally critical because it is the others who know Mr Youakim who will have to interpret his gestures. In any case, the opinions of others who know him will be vital when decisions must be made about Mr Youakim. For instance, in England and Wales, which are governed by the Mental Capacity Act (MCA), when a person lacks the capacity to make decisions about his or her care, decisions must be made in the person's best interests. The Act then specifies the people who should be consulted about the person's best interests. This includes, amongst others, 'anyone engaged in caring for the person or interested in his [sic] welfare' [MCA Section 4(7)(b)]. For Mr Youakim, this will involve his family and the carers at the home, as well as the GP and any other professionals (psychiatrists, speech and language therapists, and so on). Similar legal considerations will apply in other jurisdictions. It will almost always be the case, for instance, that family should be consulted about decisions when the person is no longer able to make decisions himself or herself. Others are important, but their opinions should also be based on their understanding of the person concerned. This understanding will increasingly depend on non-verbal gestures and other signs.

Palliative, Dementia, and Values-Based Care

Mr Youakim is now at a stage when palliative care is appropriate. It is worth being clear that the palliative care approach is relevant because it is applicable to all people with chronic, non-curable conditions. There are also palliative interventions, such as radiotherapy for pain caused by cancer which has spread to the bones. Some people, typically (but not exclusively) when nearing death, need specialist palliative care for help with complex symptom control (e.g. where syringe drivers are required).

So, if Mr Youakim now requires palliative care, does this mean that he requires a different type of care? The answer is no! First, those who are normally involved with the person should be able to provide such an approach. Second, it can be argued that the palliative care approach should, in any case, be the same as good quality, person-centred care (Hughes et al., 2006; Small et al., 2008). Thus, a palliative care approach is holistic in two senses: it involves the whole person and requires a biopsychosocial and spiritual approach, and it involves not only the person but also those around the person. But good quality person-centred dementia care should also be holistic in both of these senses.

A palliative care approach involves good communication, but so, too, does good quality, person-centred dementia care. Palliative care, like good dementia care, must involve attention to symptom control. We could even argue that there may be dementia interventions that are similar to palliative interventions. The psychosocial management of behaviours that are challenging – for instance, the use of radiotherapy for bone pain – requires a good deal of expertise, but is a targeted therapy aimed at one aspect of the bigger picture. Palliative care would try to encourage inclusion and a sense of purpose or meaning, but so, too, should good quality, person-centred care.

So, there are a variety of ways in which the palliative care approach and person-centred dementia care are the same. There are also palliative and dementia-specific interventions.

And in dementia, as in any condition, specialized palliative care may be required at some stage where complex symptoms emerge as the person approaches death. What we now wish to argue is that both the palliative care approach and good quality, person-centred dementia care are entirely in step with VBP.

For a start, understanding values is important in both palliative and dementia care. The MCA, for instance, talks about 'the beliefs and *values* that would be likely to influence his [sic] decision if he had capacity' [MCA Section 4(6)(b) emphasis added]. So, any decisions made by others in dementia or palliative care because the person is unable to make them himself or herself must take account of values. In addition, person-centredness is central to VBP, as is the multidisciplinary nature of good decision making and partnership, which are also the norm in both good quality palliative and dementia care. Similarities between palliative care, person-centred dementia care, and VBP are set out in Table 11.1.

The links between dementia and palliative care and VBP are especially obvious and important in relation to communication. And, as we have seen, communication is basic to our standing as persons.

In what follows, we shall see that different aspects of palliative care for people with dementia involve attention to both communication and values.

Advance Care Plans

Advance care planning (ACP) is something we are all encouraged to do (see Box 11.1). It makes sense. But many of us do not bother.

Table 11.1 Similarities between palliative care, person-centred dementia care, and VBP

	Palliative care	Person-centred dementia care	VBP
Understanding values	√	√	√
Person-centredness	√	√	√
Multidisciplinary approach	√	√	√
Holism	√	√	√
Good communication	√	√	√
Importance of meaning	√	√	√
Inclusion	√	√	√

Box 11.1 Definition of ACP

[A] voluntary process of discussion and review to help an individual who has capacity to anticipate how their condition may affect them in the future and, if they wish, set on record: choices about their care and treatment and/or an advance decision to refuse a treatment in specific circumstances, so that these can be referred to by those responsible for their care or treatment (whether professional staff or family carers) in the event that they lose capacity to decide once their illness progresses.

(NHS End of Life Care Programme, 2011: 6)

There is almost a policy-driven presumption that not to undertake ACP is in some sense negligent or bad. And it may be. But right at the get-go we want to say that it's a free country! After all, even if it might be sensible (and more sensible for some than others), it all depends on what we value. It can be very useful to express our own wishes or know someone else's wishes, but, equally, it's up to the individual; I might decide or another person might decide that he or she is willing to trust to fate or to the good judgement of those who might at some stage in the future have to make decisions on his or her behalf. Nevertheless, advance care planning is in step with VBP. Apart from anything else, ACP allows us to set out what is important to us, to express our values.

ACP can take a variety of forms, as shown in Box 11.2, which is based on the MCA in England and Wales. The terms will be different in other countries, but the ideas will be the same: thus, they may not be called 'Lasting Powers of Attorney', but many countries will have a system according to which a person can be nominated by someone who wants that person to be appointed to act for them if they become unable to make decisions themselves. For some examples, see Alzheimer Europe (2016).

In an ADRT you might stipulate that you do not wish to have a particular treatment under specific circumstances. This entails that you have a clear idea about the exact circumstances that might occur in the future. All you can do is refuse treatment; you cannot demand it. The person who has to put into effect your wishes has to be sure that the ADRT is valid (that you actually made it and so on) and that it is applicable (that it does clearly relate to the present circumstances). If it is valid and applicable, then it is legally binding, and it would be a violation of the law as well as potentially a criminal assault if the person was given the treatment they had refused in their ADRT. We're not going into the details of the law, because this will be different in different jurisdictions. Still, the principles will often be very similar. An ADRT (or its equivalent) allows someone with very definite views and a good deal of certainty about what might happen to convey strongly held beliefs and values. If, for instance, a man knew that he had failing kidneys and also had dementia, he might stipulate in an ADRT, whilst he still had the capacity to do so, that he would not wish to have haemodialysis for renal failure, even if not to have it would bring about his death.

It's easy to imagine in this situation how the squeaky wheel principle might come into play again. Perhaps the treating team will feel that the person has a good quality of life despite his dementia and that it is wrong to allow him to die when this seems premature. The law (at least the MCA) is clear: if the ADRT is *valid* and *applicable* then the refusal of treatment would be as if the person had refused the treatment himself with full capacity. We must abide by his decision. But perhaps the treating team will start to question its validity and applicability. Perhaps they will argue that the person could not have foreseen the current circumstances as accurately and perhaps was not fully competent (did not have full decision-making capacity) as would be required for the ADRT to be valid and

---

Box 11.2 Advance Care Planning (based on the MCA)

Advance decisions to refuse treatment (ADRTs), sometimes called Advance Directives, or Lasting Powers of Attorney (LPAs), are statements about a person's wishes, feelings, preferences, beliefs, values, etc. These may be verbal or written, but should be followed when deciding a person's best interests (and an ADRT can override best interests). These are sometimes referred to as 'values statements', (but under the MCA also have a basis in law) and for our purposes this is the terminology we shall adopt in the rest of this chapter.

applicable. VBP could usefully come into play, with attention both to the facts and values at stake, with input from all concerned, and good communication so that the process is transparent, but with the person centre stage. Using VBP might help clarify the validity and applicability of the values expressed in the ADRT. For example, were they consistent with the person's previously expressed values about illness and mortality?

LPAs in England and Wales cover both best-interests decisions concerning finance and property and welfare decisions, which can include health, social care, and housing. The donor of the powers should obviously trust the person he or she makes their decision-maker (known as the 'attorney', but this does not mean they have to be a legal professional). The basis of this trust will often be that the donor and attorney share values. Attorneys are therefore often trusted family members. It's because of the salience we attach to a person's deeply held wishes, beliefs, and values, as well as respect for the law, that practitioners should follow the instructions of the attorney. For the same reason, however, if practitioners believe that the person's wishes, beliefs, and values are not being upheld, they should challenge the attorney. In the spirit of VBP, such a challenge need not be adversarial. It would be in the spirit of trying to work out what the person concerned would value but would take into account the values being expressed by the attorney.

Of course, a values statement speaks directly to the motivations that underpin VBP. The premise of VBP, remember, is **mutual respect for differences of value**. A values statement also accepts as a premise that people may have different values, which is why they may need to be set out clearly. In law, such a statement has very little weight, in the sense that it cannot compel particular treatments and is not an ADRT. But morally, if your values are clearly stated and known, it is hard to ignore them and, under the MCA at least, they must be considered in trying to determine what might be in your best interests if you are unable to make decisions for yourself.

Mr Youakim, like many people, had made a power of attorney when he was first diagnosed to cover finances and property in favour of his two children who lived in England but not to cover welfare issues to do with his health. He had neither written an ADRT nor a values statement, partly because he'd not heard of them.

Vignette - Mr Youakim (2): Use of Antibiotics

Mr Youakim has already suffered a series of chest infections. He develops a further infection. When the GP comes to see him, he is almost unresponsive. He has a high fever, and there are sounds in his chest which are in keeping with a severe chest infection. He will still take little sips of water, but his eyes are shut and he is short of breath. He looks a deathly colour.

The GP, Dr Gilchrist, discusses matters with the staff. They say that they know that Mr Youakim's daughter, Marie, who lives locally, would not want her father to be admitted to hospital. When this had happened previously, the whole experience had been profoundly distressing for him. Marie arrives at the home whilst Dr Gilchrist is still there. They discuss what should be done. Dr Gilchrist is frank: her father could die, and the best chance for him to survive would be for him to be admitted to hospital to receive intravenous antibiotics. Marie expresses her concerns about her father going into hospital, and the staff agree and say that they want to care for him in the home, because they know him well. They also point out, and Marie agrees, that of late Mr Youakim has seemed quite content and even happy, despite his deteriorated physical state. Dr Gilchrist says that she fully understands and agrees too. She suggests that it might be possible to treat him with an oral antibiotic in the home if he will tolerate it and swallow it as a liquid. He can also be given some paracetamol in soluble form to lower his temperature and keep him comfortable. She asks Marie what she thinks her father would have wanted. Marie doesn't know: they never discussed this sort of thing. She asks if she can ring her brother, Spiro. He says that he thinks their father was fairly fatalistic and would have accepted the inevitability of death. He agrees with the plan not to admit Mr Youakim, but says he also feels it may be a waste of effort giving him the antibiotics by mouth. He speaks to Dr Gilchrist, and they agree, nonetheless, that it is worth trying the oral antibiotics, as long as this does not cause Mr Youakim distress. The staff say they are very happy to try giving the antibiotic, because they would otherwise feel that they were just watching him die when perhaps they could have done something for him. It's decided, therefore, to give him oral antibiotics and paracetamol in liquid form for a few days to see how he does.

Without stretching the point too far, it can be seen that the process of VBP is entirely appropriate to the scenario we have just sketched. In Table 11.2 we have set out briefly the components of the ten-part process of VBP and shown how the different parts of the process relate to Mr Youakim's story so far.

Eating and Drinking

One quick point to note is that in the medical and medical ethics literature, eating and drinking in the contexts we are considering are often referred to as 'artificial nutrition and hydration' (ANH). It's easy not to notice that this positions the process as a medical one. It helps to make it a technical issue: he can't swallow, so he needs ANH, and the best way to do this (it might be and has often been argued) is with a percutaneous endoscopic gastrostomy (PEG) tube, which, as we discussed in Chapter 9, is a tube inserted directly through the abdominal wall into the stomach. Food and fluid can then be put straight into the stomach without much inconvenience.

There is a logic to all of this, but it takes us some way from the everyday notions of eating and drinking. Eating and drinking occur in various forms and play a significant role in our lives. We use food and drink to celebrate important milestones in our lives: birthdays, anniversaries, and so on. And although we can eat on our own, eating and drinking are often used as a means to come together socially. ANH and PEG feeding are decidedly not social occasions. The very terminology holds evaluative connotations. But let's return to Mr Youakim.

Vignette - Mr Youakim (3): PEG Feeding

Mr Youakim gradually improved. The care staff were able to get him to take the antibiotic on most occasions that it was due, and his improvement seemed to follow. Everyone was very relieved. He was returning to his old self, still entirely dependent and unable to communicate verbally, but nonetheless able to demonstrate his basic likes and dislikes.

Dr Gilchrist was pleased that things seemed to have worked out well. She then received an email from Mr Youakim's other daughter, Ava, who lives abroad. Ava thanked Dr Gilchrist for the personal interest she had taken in her father's care, but she said she was concerned about the frequent infections her father was getting, especially because

Table 11.2 Mr Youakim and the ten-part process of values-based practice

Ten-part process of VBP		Mr Youakim's story
Four areas of clinical skill	Awareness of values	Dr Gilchrist is aware that she needs to allow people to express their concerns, which reflect their values, and she notes a slight discrepancy between what Marie and Spiro have said. He has said that his father would be 'fatalistic'.
	Reasoning	In her judgements about Mr Youakim, Dr Gilchrist is able to draw upon her knowledge of other cases (i.e. she is using the approach of casuistry). If his chest infection were a little more severe, e.g. if he were completely unable to take anything by mouth, she would not even have raised the question of an admission to hospital on the grounds that it might then have been possible to say that he was definitely dying. But she cannot say this: the prognosis is uncertain. So steering a middle course and making a decision that could be reversed seems sensible in this case.
	Knowledge	By chance, Dr Gilchrist had recently attended a refresher course on dementia at the Royal College of General Practitioners. A speaker on palliative care and dementia had mentioned the work of a team from The Netherlands who had shown that decisions about whether or not to treat chest infections in advanced dementia can be quite nuanced: a decision can be made not to use antibiotics at all; or they can be used with curative intent; or they might be used in a palliative fashion to try to settle symptoms (van der Steen et al., 2002). Knowing that this is a possibility had been helpful in Dr Gilchrist's decision making.
	Communication	Clearly Dr Gilchrist was willing to listen to everyone involved in Mr Youakim's care and she felt it was important that Spiro was involved in the decision. She had tried to be straightforward in her communications with them. She had a good relationship with the care home staff and felt she could rely on their judgements. They knew her well enough to feel able to speak their minds and express their feelings.
Relationships	Person-centred practice	Throughout the decision making, Mr Youakim had been the focus of their attention. Little was really known about how he would have felt, except he was said to be fatalistic. If he had made a relevant advance care plan, they might have known more. But as it is, he did appoint Marie and Spiro to be his attorneys for matters related to money. So he obviously valued their opinions. He was situated in his family – they remain close and involved – so focusing on him does not preclude involving them as key players in decisions about him.
	Multi-disciplinary teamwork	The different disciplines involved in his care have been able to express their views. Both the nurses and the care assistants in the home, who know him well, seem to agree. Dr Gilchrist also benefits from knowing the views of her District Nursing colleagues who have been in to see Mr Youakim several times over the last few weeks.
Evidence and values	The two-feet principle	It is also very clear in this case that both facts and values are at play. But despite a thorough clinical examination, a value judgement has still been required about treatment.
	The squeaky wheel principle	Dr Gilchrist senses that Spiro and Marie are making slightly different evaluative judgements when it comes to their father. Marie did not wish him to be admitted to hospital but obviously wanted him to be treated. Spiro seemed less set on the idea that treatment should be pursued, as long as his father was comfortable.
	The science-driven principle	In the background, Dr Gilchrist was aware that the hospital would be able to keep Mr Youakim alive. At an extreme – not one that anyone was suggesting – he could be taken to intensive care and ventilated until a strong enough antibiotic was found to treat his infection. The possibility of invasive treatments has inevitably increased the need for evaluative judgements, not decreased them.
Partnership	Consensus or dissensus	They had arrived at a consensus today, although Spiro's talk of fatalism was noted. It would have to be seen how things would play out subsequently.

this most recent one had been so bad. Her local friends who have experience with dementia told her that in their country her father would have a PEG tube by now so that his food would not go down into his lungs, which is what she is guessing must be happening. She's visiting in two weeks and wants to have a meeting with Dr Gilchrist.

It's decided to have a full family and multidisciplinary meeting. Marie is, of course, present, but Spiro also comes down. Dr Gilchrist gives a quick summary of what's been happening medically, and the care home staff also bring the family up to date. Ava raises the issue of the PEG tube immediately and says she understands it will help to stop chest infections, make it less likely that their father will get pressure sores, and will stop him from losing weight, which has been a worry. Marie says she thinks it sounds like a good idea and wonders why it's not been done before. But Spiro says he thinks their father would have hated the idea and that his view is that nature should take its course. This upsets both Ava and Marie, but Spiro says they have to be realistic, to which they retort that he's being callous. The care staff are rather on Spiro's side and think that fitting a feeding tube would be terrible for Mr Youakim, partly because this would mean a hospital admission. Hearing this makes Marie think again, but she is torn between her wish to avoid a further hospital visit for her father and her inclination to do something that will stop him from getting ill.

Dr Gilchrist then steps in to thank everyone for offering their views. She acknowledges that there are a number of things (reflecting their values) that they have in common: they all want the best for Mr Youakim; they all want to avoid him harm; they want to do what he would have wanted them to do. She is then able to set out some facts about PEG tubes, which she has researched, knowing that the issue was going to arise. She summarizes a Cochrane Review (Sampson et al., 2009) which found that there was insufficient evidence to suggest this type of tube feeding is beneficial in advanced dementia. Ava finds this hard to accept given that PEG tubes are used so frequently in the country where she is living. Dr Gilchrist acknowledges that different countries see things differently – they express different values – but is able to point out that the view that most adopt in the UK is shared by many other countries and that awareness of the lack of good evidence about the effectiveness of PEG tubes (at least in advanced dementia) is spreading. She also points out that potential harms are associated with PEG tubes, from infections to bleeding.

She asks them to focus on what they think Mr Youakim would want for himself. It's agreed that he was not particularly keen on medical interventions: he was always happy to let things fix themselves. Spiro again says he thinks their father was fatalistic, which is how he seemed when he spoke about other people in the family who were ill.

Ava remains a little sceptical that a PEG tube would not be a way to stop food going into the lungs. She's slightly swayed when it's explained that material can still ascend from the stomach and oesophagus to go down the trachea, which might then be a source of infection. The care home team talk about how they will implement the advice of the speech and language therapists and ensure that Mr Youakim has the right posture and the right consistency of food. This appeases Ava. She says she trusts the staff, but she says she'd like to get a second opinion, which Dr Gilchrist is happy to arrange. There appears to be a consensus, although the concerns of Ava have been noted and will be further addressed.

What we see here are the elements of VBP in action: awareness of values, the use of facts and reasoning, good communication, person-centred practice within a multidisciplinary setting, and the importance of facts and values – both shared and diverse values – with a degree of consensus and dissensus.

Vignette - Mr Youakim (4): Resuscitation

The meeting moved on to consider resuscitation. Spiro said that he doesn't think their father is enjoying a good quality of life. The care staff in the home responded that he does sometimes smile. Marie agreed and said that if Spiro visited more frequently he would see this. Dr Gilchrist said that because it's always difficult to judge someone else's quality of life, it is perhaps better to think about whether a treatment (or an investigation) is (1) likely to be effective and (2) likely to be burdensome for the person, as well as for his or her family. In the case of cardiopulmonary resuscitation (CPR) in people with advanced dementia, she says, the chances of a successful resuscitation in a care home are quite remote, so it's unlikely to be effective (Finucane and Harper, 1999). In addition, she says, the process of CPR is undignified, can lead to harm (e.g. broken ribs), and might leave him in a worse state than he is already. On these grounds CPR could be considered burdensome. Dr Gilchrist feels, therefore, that there is no moral obligation to undertake CPR and she invites the family to give their views. Spiro is clear it is the last thing their father would want. Ava says that there is no point in doing something that's going to be futile. Marie says she'd not want to see her father suffer any more, but she'd still want other things to be treated if they could be. The care staff are sympathetic, but say they will need all of this to be documented and signed; otherwise, they'd be duty-bound to try to resuscitate Mr Youakim. The meeting ended on a sad note but with some unanimity.

Once again, we see VBP being put into effect. People are encouraged to express their views, and there is consensus, even if there is some divergence in terms of what people value the most. But the broader point we wish to make is that if this is a good example of VBP in action, it is also a good example of both good quality dementia care and good palliative care. Furthermore, a central feature of all of this is good communication. And this will inevitably be important if we are person-centred.

European Association of Palliative Care White Paper

None of this should be a surprise to those who work in the field of palliative care and dementia. In 2014, a white paper was published on behalf of the European Association of Palliative Care which defined optimal palliative care for people with dementia (van der Steen et al., 2014). A number of their recommendations are completely in keeping with VBP. For example:

> 2.1 Perceived problems in caring for a patient with dementia should be viewed from the patient's perspective, applying the concept of person-centred care.

> 2.2 Shared decision making includes the patient and family caregiver as partners and is an appealing model that should be aimed for.

...

> 2.5 Current or previously expressed preferences with regard to place of care should be honoured as a principle, but best interest, safety and family caregiver burden issues should also be given weight in decisions on place of care.

> 2.6 Within the multidisciplinary team, patient and family issues should be discussed on a regular basis.

(van der Steen et al., 2014)

In connection with advance care planning, the white paper was clear and overtly stressed the role of values:

> 3.2 Anticipating progression of the disease, advance care planning is proactive. This implies it should start as soon as the diagnosis is made, when the patient can still be actively involved *and patient preferences, values, needs and beliefs can be elicited*'
> (van der Steen et al., 2014, emphasis added)

Good communication, palliative care, person-centred dementia care, and VBP coalesce. The premise of VBP – mutual respect for differences of values – is central to all these approaches. Good communication allows and accepts the expression of diverse values. Recognizing and understanding such values is essential to good quality care, whether such care is provided through the lens of practitioners in palliative care or dementia care.

Back to the Manifesto

The focus of this chapter has been communication, and we have devoted it to the subject of palliative care for people living with dementia. This seems natural enough because palliative care is one of the fields of clinical practice (along with general practice and psychiatry) where there has long been a heavy emphasis placed on the importance of good communication. This emphasis has spread, and now communication skills training plays an important part in the education of all doctors, as it has done for some time in the training of nurses and other allied health and social care professionals. However, not everyone thinks this is an unequivocal good. The philosopher Robin Downie, writing in *Advances in Psychiatric Treatment*, says this:

> The very term 'communication skills' is the giveaway in that it suggests that there are generalisable skills that are teachable and learnable and, therefore, widely applicable. Perhaps there are, but they are unlikely to extend much beyond such matters as avoiding technical terms, not speaking too quickly, repeating the message and so on. These things are, of course, of the first importance because a common criticism of doctors generally is that they are deficient in such matters. Nevertheless, attempts to have a complete reduction of communication to a set of discrete skills is bound to fail. Patients and their problems and psychiatrists and their personalities are all too varied for any reductionist approach to work. Indeed, interaction with patients may be adversely affected if trainee psychiatrists are encouraged to inhibit their own natural responses and substitute consciously adopted trained responses (Randall [and Downie], 2006). Human communication will become a manipulative technique.
> (Downie, 2012)

Now it might be that we should not be so disparaging about communication skills training. There's no reason why such training should not furnish a person with both mundane skills and higher skills of the sort that Downie would approve. As one of us (JCH) said in a commentary in response to Downie:

> Any dullard can quickly acquire the vocabulary of architectural appreciation (e.g. flying buttresses, fan vaulting, Ionic capitals), but it is also possible to learn how to attend (to acquire the skills), so that we see or hear in a way that is more informed

and more reflective. Of course, there is something else – to do with aptitude, temperament and experience – that means that some of us will always find good communication difficult ... The point, it seems, is not to disparage the possibility of acquiring higher skills, but to ponder their nature and how they are acquired. It might be by example, but then, I suspect, what is acquired is not some mere skill: rather, an attitude or way of life.

(Hughes, 2012)

Downie was, however, addressing an important clinical point. Good communication is a matter of far more importance than the simple acquisition of some skills. It's also an important philosophical point:

Downie is correct to commend 'engaged attention'. Our day-to-day experience of this is, I think, more than an experience of both the human and scientific sides of medicine. It is an experience of the mundane, but the mundane, the everyday, presupposes shared commitments – meanings, values, intuitions, emotions and so forth – that can never be fully specified; nonetheless, they are implicit in clinical practice.

(Hughes, 2012)

This debate is relevant to dementia and fits in with the first principle of our Manifesto. Communication is an important ingredient of VBP and it is relevant to dementia care, not just in the severe stages of dementia, when it is more challenging, but right from the start (e.g. when ACP is contemplated). We need good, clear communication. This is not required, however, because the person has dementia. It is required because, as human beings in the world, it is both essential for instrumental reasons (i.e. it helps us to get things done) and quintessential in that it defines us as human beings. The importance of information being communicated in accessible ways is also a right under Article 9 of the United Nations Convention on the Rights of Persons with Disabilities (UNCRPD), as well as in some national laws. Even people living with advanced dementia deserve clarity of communication because it might be helpful. Clear communication might help them to understand what is about to happen. But they also deserve clear communication just because they are people like the rest of us. Of course, communication is not just a matter of what we say. We also communicate non-verbally, which can reflect emotional states (positive or negative) and elicit emotional responses (positive or negative). Our attitudes towards people who live with dementia – shown by how we communicate with them – reflect our basic humanity.

Dementia is a unique touchstone for understanding the human condition.

Meanwhile, VBP, which incorporates good communication as an essential clinical skill, provides a framework for good care. It allows us to handle difficult situations – for instance, at the end of life – with a degree of confidence knowing that, if we stick to the approach of VBP, we shall deal with people fairly and respect their right to self-determination insofar as this is possible. The second principle of the Manifesto reflects this basic point.

Dementia as a disability and a disease emphasizes the rights of people living with dementia to all the normal benefits of citizenship.

The process of caring for someone like Mr Youakim is governed by laws, which are designed to uphold his rights. He is still a citizen. But it is not just a legal process, it's also one that is in keeping with the process of VBP. Communication is part of this, but it's more than that, because it defines the whole way in which we are with each other. We can *be with* people in ways that show we are not really interested in them, or we can *be with* them – as Dr Gilchrist is – in ways which show our concern and solicitude (Hughes, 2011: 47–48). Meanwhile, the third principle of the Manifesto is also in evidence: attentive listening to the words of the family and all those involved in Mr Youakim's care elicits their values and allows a meaningful exchange so that all can feel they have been heard. This is supportive, but it is also the right way to treat people. At the same time, the palpable effects of Mr Youakim's dementia on his body's ability to perform basic functions reminds us that expert, professional care and treatment are still essential to deal with the disease aspects of the condition.

VBP and an awareness of rights provide an essential framework for providing support, care, and treatment to people with dementia, their families, and their friends.

Attention to their values shows respect for persons. Taking account of the values of all concerned is also just one way of demonstrating how VBP provides a framework. It need not be explicit, but when values are engaged, conversations are often more straightforward. People who understand VBP will, by inclination, be alert to values and to divergent values that need to be addressed. Allowing everyone to have their say in a manner and environment in which they feel they have been heard is another important way in which to enthuse and interact with all concerned in the person's care. Involving others becomes more critical as the person living with dementia becomes less able to represent himself or herself. This 'engaged attention' to the person living with dementia is also a means by which to ensure that his or her rights are upheld and not ignored. Taking a rights-based approach is another way to allow people living with dementia to flourish in a world where they might otherwise be ignored. 'VBP plus rights' emphasizes the importance of the standing of the person with dementia. It is not solely that they have values, but even where these are obscured by cognitive impairment, they also have rights to certain sorts of treatment (social as well as clinical), as well as legal protections.

Conclusion

People living with dementia are persons from start to finish (Hughes, 2001). Communication is important to people living with dementia, as it is to all of us, for important instrumental and conceptual reasons. It is central to VBP, but is also crucial for good quality, person-centred dementia care, and this is no more apparent than towards the end of life when good communication forms part of the palliative care approach. From a different perspective, that of human rights, good communication also means hearing the voices of people with dementia. To the VBP framework we wish to add a human rights framework. In order to respect the values of people with dementia, we need recognition of their basic human rights.

In an incisive paper on disability and dementia, Shakespeare et al. (2017) have suggested that 'a relational model of dementia lays the basis for a human rights approach to the condition'. They argue that

> it is vital to situate the individual experience of dementia in the broader social context. We also need to articulate a human rights perspective in which self-advocacy is core. We need

to expand our ideas about social models and about human rights in order to incorporate the experience of all human beings, including people living with dementia.

(Shakespeare et al., 2017)

The person living with dementia is a person with values, but is also a person with rights which must be respected throughout his or her life. Communication is key, but it is not just communicating *to* the person, it is communicating *with* them, and with those who maintain the person's standing as a self in a social context. It is a duty for all concerned: to hear the voices of people living with dementia.

> If we are beginning to understand the voice that people with dementia retain, and the possibilities for a more expanded understanding of personhood, then we open the doors to a more powerful articulation of the rights of people with dementia and thus their ability to retain their humanity to the end of their lives.
>
> (Shakespeare et al., 2017)

Key points

- There are a number of ways in which communication can be facilitated for people with dementia, but this remains challenging when dementia is more advanced.
- Our abilities to communicate have an impact on our standing as persons or human beings: communication is part and parcel of our humanity.
- Person-centred dementia care, palliative care, and VBP embrace the same elements of care, and good quality communication is vital to all three approaches.
- The links between the three approaches to care are seen in a variety of issues that arise in advanced dementia, for example, advance care planning, the use of antibiotics, eating and drinking, and resuscitation.
- Communication is essential to our ability to work together, but it is quintessential to our being as persons. This is true of all of us, as it is for people with dementia.
- But it is not just about communicating *to* people living with dementia, it is also about communicating *with* them and, crucially, it is about hearing the voice of people with dementia.
- Underpinning the duty to hear the voice of people with dementia is not only our common humanity, but also the human rights that flow from that shared standing as people with values.

References

Allan, K., and Killick, J. (2010). Communicating with people with dementia. Ch 23 in J. C. Hughes, M. Lloyd-Williams, and G. A. Sachs, eds., *Supportive Care for the Person with Dementia*. Oxford: Oxford University Press, pp. 217–25.

Alzheimer Europe. (2016). *Dementia in Europe Yearbook 2016. Decision Making and Legal Capacity in Dementia*. Luxembourg: Alzheimer Europe.

Downie, R. (2012). Paying attention: Hippocratic and Asklepian approaches. *Advances in Psychiatric Treatment* 18, 363–68.

Ellis, M., and Astell, A. J. (2017). *Adaptive Interaction and Dementia: How to Communicate Without Speech*. London and Philadelphia: Jessica Kingsley.

Finucane, T. E., and Harper, G. M. (1999). Attempting resuscitation in nursing homes: Policy considerations. *Journal of the American Geriatric Society* 47(10), 1261–64.

Hughes, J. C. (2001). Views of the person with dementia. *Journal of Medical Ethics* 27, 86–91.

(2011). *Thinking Through Dementia*. Oxford: Oxford University Press.

(2012). Searching for real holism. Commentary on … paying attention. *Advances in Psychiatric Treatment*, 18, 369–71.

Hughes, J. C., Hedley K., and Harris, D. (2006). The practice and philosophy of palliative care in dementia. In Hughes, J. C., ed., *Palliative Care in Severe Dementia*. London: Quay Books, pp. 1–11.

Killick, J., and Allan, K. (2001). *Communication and the Care of People with Dementia*. Buckingham: Open University Press.

Murphy, J., and Oliver, T. M. (2013). The use of Talking Mats to support people with dementia and their carers to make decisions together. *Health & Social Care in the Community* 21(2), 171–80.

NHS National End of Life Care Programme. (2011). *Capacity, Care Planning and Advance Care Planning in Life Limiting Illness: A Guide for Health and Social Care Staff*. Available via: www.ncpc.org.uk/ sites/default/files/ACP_Booklet_June_2011 .pdf [Last accessed: 25 November 2017]

Randall, F., and Downie, R. (2006). *The Philosophy of Palliative Care: Critique and Re-Construction*. Oxford: Oxford University Press.

Sabat, S. R. (2001). *The Experience of Alzheimer's Disease: Life Through a Tangled Veil*. Oxford and Malden, MA: Blackwell.

Sampson, E. L., Candy, B., and Jones, L. (2009). Enteral tube feeding for older people with advanced dementia. *Cochrane Database Systematic Review*. April 15(2):CD007209. doi: 10.1002/14651858.CD007209.pub2. [Last accessed: 1 December 2017].

Shakespeare, T., Zeilig, H., and Mittler, P. (2017). Rights in mind: Thinking differently about dementia and disability. *Dementia* 0(0), 1–14. doi: 10.1177/1471301217701506

Small, N., Froggatt, K., and Downs, M. (2008). *Living and Dying with Dementia: Dialogues about Palliative Care*. Oxford: Oxford University Press.

van der Steen, J. T., Ooms, M. E., Mehr, D. R., et al. (2002). Severe dementia and adverse outcomes of nursing home-acquired pneumonia: Evidence for mediation by functional and pathophysiological decline. *Journal of the American Geriatrics Society* 50, 439–48.

van der Steen, J. T., Radbruch, L., Hertogh, C. M. P. M., et al. (2014). White paper defining optimal palliative care in older people with dementia: A Delphi study and recommendations from the European Association for Palliative Care. *Palliative Medicine* 28(3), 197–209.

Chapter 12

Partnerships in Decision Making

Topics covered in this chapter
- Values are expressed implicitly and explicitly through partnerships and in decision making.
- Partnerships are important in dementia care, ranging from the relationship with a person with dementia through to the notion of solidarity at a societal level.
- Practice, ethics, and the law locate decision making in the individual; dementia challenges this, but concepts such as shared and supported decision making and relational autonomy can address this challenge.
- The framework provided by dissensus can be applied in situations where there are differences in values.
- Dissensus can give people a more inclusive perspective, as well as the means to make decisions and take action involving all the values and rights 'in play' in particular situations in dementia care.

Take-away message for practice
Forming and sustaining partnerships with the person with dementia, carers, and a range of practitioners is vital in dementia care, especially around decision making. Consensus may not always be achievable or desirable, especially where a person with dementia has difficulty making decisions, but dissensus (which is not the same as disagreement) provides a way of ensuring all the relevant values and rights are taken into account.

Introduction

The last element of the VBP process puts the spotlight on partnership and specifically the importance of partnership in decision making. Over time, day-to-day decision making about people's care and treatment in health and social care has moved from a position where professionals frequently made or directed decisions – "doctor knows best" – to a more collaborative, shared decision-making approach with service users and carers. Partnership in decision making therefore may seem fairly straightforward and self-explanatory. But VBP recognizes that in many situations a collaborative and consensual approach to decision making isn't always possible because of differences in values. VBP aims to address this through the concept of 'dissensus' – a positive and constructive approach to disagreements involving values.

This chapter explores how partnership in decision making can be applied in dementia care and how it relates to the principles of our Manifesto. It identifies some tensions that can exist between practice focused on values underpinning partnership and values underpinning decision-making processes. The chapter describes different values and approaches that can bring partnership and decision making together, taking into account the effect dementia has on a person's ability to make decisions: their mental capacity. But bringing partnership and decision making together does not prevent differences in people's values leading to disagreements. The chapter describes in several different ways how 'dissensus' can be helpful when disagreements in dementia care arise and how this links with the principles of our Manifesto.

To understand partnership in decision making and the concept of dissensus in relation to dementia, we will consider each component separately.

Partnerships

'Partnership' suggests collaboration and agreement; consensus over shared values, decisions, and actions. While we have drawn attention to situations in dementia care where there are differences in values, for many people these differences do not occur. Agreement between the person with dementia, professionals, and carers may well occur about the diagnosis of dementia; the best options for care, support, and treatment; and the need for a move into residential care (although it may be harder to discern the real wishes of the person with dementia regarding the latter). In these situations VBP is less relevant because there is consensus.

Consensus requires little explanation. Consensus is built around an agreement about the best decision or course of action based on all the relevant evidence. It is intrinsic to evidence-based practice (EBP) and can almost be a scientific process by which other options are ruled out because the evidence does not support them. Partnerships based on consensus are therefore straightforward, except that there must still exist the right environment in which to allow such consensus to emerge.

Where VBP becomes useful is where consensus within partnerships cannot be achieved because the partnership involves people with a range of values, conflicting values, or uncertainty about values. The premise of VBP is mutual respect for different values, so it does not exclude values on the basis of them being right or wrong, as compared with facts which are either correct or incorrect based upon scientific evidence (although how evidence is gathered and used can depend upon judgements involving values). Consensus can be reached around a diagnosis of vascular dementia through an assessment process involving a magnetic resonance imaging (MRI) scan. But someone making the choice not to seek a diagnosis is doing something that is factually neither correct nor incorrect, even if facts are involved; the decision is based upon the person's values and includes their right to make such decisions. Consensus may therefore not be achievable, and although the person might subsequently change his or her mind, consensus may not be a framework that a partnership can use. Similarly, an assessment of the driving ability and safety of a person with dementia may clearly show that they must no longer drive. But driving is often a very important part of a person's identity and status. So although the person may accept the facts of the assessment, they may be profoundly unhappy and not part of the consensus (say between the family and the doctor) that agrees on the outcome.

Consensus may be desirable but must either be negotiated or alternatives sought, depending upon the particularities of each situation.

Let's consider in more detail some aspects of partnership where values diversity arises.

Partnership and Communication

In the previous chapter we discussed the importance of communicating *with* the person with dementia, not just *to* them. This is vital in order to understand the values that are informing their behaviour, decisions, and actions. We also flagged up the difficulties that can arise in communicating with people with dementia and various ways of overcoming these difficulties, through the involvement of others and/or the use of particular communication systems. Meaningful communication requires partnership.

A simple but important example of this involves people with intellectual disabilities (also referred to as learning disabilities) who develop dementia, which is very common. People with more severe intellectual disabilities may have only limited verbal communication or be unable to communicate verbally at all. This can make it very difficult for them to express what's important to them – their values – and for others to know what these are.

A range of communication systems have been developed for people with intellectual disabilities, ranging from the use of picture symbols (Frost and Bondy, 1994) to an approach called 'intensive interaction' (Firth and Barber, 2011), which the adaptive interaction approach for dementia, described in Chapter 11, is based upon. Diagnosing dementia and providing appropriate care and support to people with intellectual disabilities can be particularly challenging for dementia practitioners. Forming partnerships with family members and intellectual disabilities services that are familiar with these specialist types of communication is therefore essential. Similarly, for people with dementia from Black, Asian, and minority ethnic groups, issues of language, terminology, and cultural expressions that may describe or be underpinned by their values require partnerships with experts in these areas.

Partnership with the Person with Dementia

Forming positive, collaborative partnerships in is an essential skill in health and social care. The 'doctor–patient relationship', 'service user engagement', and 'therapeutic relationship' are all common terms denoting this notion of partnership in everyday practice. Research and professional experience consistently tell us that it is the quality of the relationship between a practitioner and service user that is as good an indicator of how successful or sustained therapeutic interventions will be, including concordance with treatment, as the intervention or treatment itself.[1] Of course, there are inequalities in this partnership involving diverse values because of differences in lived experience, professional expertise, knowledge, and power, which can all affect the relationship. VBP's emphasis on understanding and being open and aware of these values is crucial in trying to ensure these differences do not affect the partnership in unhelpful or negative ways.

---

[1] There are numerous studies about the importance and effectiveness of the therapeutic relationship in mental health care, but this is a relatively unexplored area in dementia care. For more general studies see for example, Luker et al. (2000); McCabe and Priebe (2004); Reynolds (2009) (especially pp. 317–18).

This book has provided numerous examples of partnerships in dementia care and highlighted the particular challenges that dementia can pose in forming and sustaining partnerships. If a person does not know they have dementia, denies it, chooses not to disclose it, is unaware, or can't remember its effects, a partnership in decision making about care and treatment with a practitioner becomes more difficult. As we saw in the last chapter with Mr Youakim, and with other examples we have given, the progression of dementia makes it more and more difficult for a person with the condition to communicate and for those around the person to know exactly what they are experiencing. But the onus must still be on practitioners doing all they can to form and maintain a partnership with the person with dementia regarding the person's care and treatment. What's important to the person with dementia – their values – must guide the partnership and form the basis of the decision-making process. This is the essence of person-centred practice described in Chapter 6 and is aligned with our principles of dementia as humanity and with a disease model or a disability model view of dementia. But while person-centred practice, focused on the individual with dementia, should be the cornerstone in dementia care, the parameters of partnership usually have to be expanded to include others.

Here it is worth noting that many people with dementia live alone; in the UK, it has been estimated that as many as one-third of people with dementia live alone (Miranda-Castillo et al., 2010). This can create particular challenges for practitioners to develop useful and meaningful partnerships, especially because many people with dementia living alone will be in residential care and severely impaired by their dementia. It highlights the importance of encouraging and supporting people with dementia to make their wishes, feelings, beliefs, values, preferences, and dislikes clear before they lose the ability to do so. Chapter 11 gave some examples of ways of doing this.

Partnership with Others

In Chapters 6 and 7, we discussed how different values can be expressed and worked within the context of family relationships and multidisciplinary working. The majority of people with dementia will have experienced a range of relationships in their lives and will have at least one family member (usually a husband, wife, partner, or spouse) they continue to live with while they remain in their own home. These relationships are intimate, emotional (not always in a positive sense), and deeply personal. While 'carer' denotes a specific role in relation to a person with dementia, the family member who occupies this role may not wish to define themselves as a carer, and it certainly does not define the totality of their relationship with the person with dementia. Concepts such as 'relationship-centred care' and the 'triangle of care' draw attention to the importance of recognizing the role and values of family members in dementia care (see Chapter 6).

Partnership also involves recognizing the role of other 'players' who can make important contributions to the care of people with dementia. This includes people such as staff working in primary care and general hospitals; social care staff such as social workers; staff working in care homes and those providing domiciliary care; people working or volunteering for non-profit and voluntary organizations such as dementia advisors, support workers, and advocates; organizations working with people with dementia from 'seldom-heard groups' described in Chapter 10; and supported housing staff, welfare benefits advisors, employers, and legal professionals; as well as others with dementia through peer support initiatives (Chakkalackal, 2014).

In Chapter 7, we discussed staff working together and multidisciplinary teams (MDTs); clearly partnerships between different practitioners are vital. This must involve an understanding of the professional values that practitioners bring to dementia care from their disciplines (e.g. doctors, nurses, psychologists, social workers, etc.) but also the different values that their organizations have (e.g. health care, social care). Because of the physical effects of dementia as well as the likelihood of co-morbidities, partnerships also have to be formed with a variety of other health and social care services through collaborative working or integrated services. Useful summaries of the evidence for the benefits of multidisciplinary teams and the importance of forming collaborative partnerships between disciplines and services, including carers and care homes, can be found in Adams et al. (2003); Struble et al. (2013, especially pp. 79–85); and Thompsell (2011).

But as we saw with Mr Youakim in the last chapter, all these other players bring their own values, which may or may not be aligned. Decision making about percutaneous endoscopic gastrostomy (PEG) feeding and palliative care for Mr Youakim involved his son and daughters, the GP, care home staff, a speech and language therapist, and potentially other health care professionals who might be asked to insert a PEG tube. Positive partnership working had to be created and sustained with all these people. Although the facts of the situation were relatively clear, there were choices to be made and therefore values had to be considered as well. Remember the adage in Chapter 8 (and its inverse in Chapter 9): 'think facts; think values'. Added to this is the importance of at least one person in the partnership being aware of how rights may apply in certain situations.

Furthermore, in some ways Mr Youakim's situation was relatively simple in terms of how many people were involved in the partnership. Barbara Pointon, a well-known family carer from the UK who has spoken widely about caring for her husband, Malcolm, who had Alzheimer's disease, has frequently used a diagram (Figure 12.1) to illustrate the bewildering array of people involved in Malcolm's care in the last seven years of his life.

Of course, not all the people in the diagram would be involved in every situation or partnership where a decision was being made about Malcolm's care. But all had to form partnerships with Barbara and Malcolm, and with others, and VBP would suggest that they should understand each other's values when making decisions. 'Too much!' you may say! And Barbara Pointon uses the diagram to argue for a single source of expert advice in the form of a trained dementia nurse. In some countries specialist nurses performing a similar role do exist, such as Admiral Nurses in the UK.[2] A role such as this certainly has its benefits but does not preclude the need for other practitioners to be involved. So the importance of partnership remains.

Yet as the first principle of the Manifesto suggests, we believe that dementia care also needs to recognize partnership in an even wider context. Dementia as humanity directs our attention to the experience of people with dementia as members of communities and society, citizens of a *polis*, but also the very essence of what it is to be human. It is worth at this point taking a brief diversion into the most common theory of evolution.

Although attention to the work of Charles Darwin has often focused on notions of competition and natural selection, Darwin also recognized how cooperation and interdependency appeared to be an intrinsic part of animal and human behaviour. Humans

---

[2] Admiral Nurses are qualified nurses with specialist training and support provided by a voluntary-sector organization, Dementia UK: www.dementiauk.org.

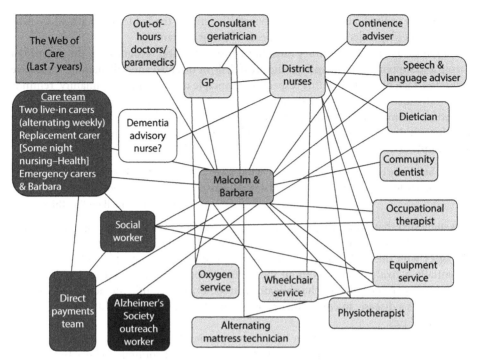

Figure 12.1 The 'Web of Care'
[Reproduced with the kind permission of Barbara Pointon]

and many other species have complex social and ecological systems, and some have argued that humans are 'eusocial': considered to be the highest level of organization of animal sociality based on cooperation and a clear division of labour (most commonly associated with ants, termites, wasps, and bees). Certainly human social systems, whether advanced capitalism or the few hunter-gatherer societies that still exist, rely upon vast amounts of cooperative behaviour and role differentiation. As an interesting aside, the Russian nineteenth-century anarchist philosopher Peter Kropotkin challenged prevailing notions of interpersonal competition and natural hierarchy based upon an interpretation of Darwin's work and argued that mutual aid was crucial to the survival of human and animal communities.

More recently, the philosopher Mary Midgley has, in her book *The Solitary Self*, made the same point about the social aspects of Darwin's writings. Concerning *Homo sapiens*, she writes: 'Like other social animals, they are not shaped for heroic solitude but for profound cooperation with others, living interdependently in friendly association' (Midgley, 2010: 24). Towards the end of the book she suggests 'that other people are constantly present to us and must always be considered, so that mutual influence continually flows between us' (Midgley, 2010: 140).

Strict evolutionists might refer to the notion of 'survival of the fittest' and point to how different species treat members who are old and ill by ostracizing them. A shift from the ideology of collectivism, which developed in many countries through the twentieth century and gave rise to publicly provided health, housing, and welfare systems, towards an emphasis on individualism in the late twentieth century tended to focus attention away from the interdependent and social aspects of being human.

Yet in the twenty-first century most human societies still recognize the importance of caring and supporting its members who are old, ill, or disabled and still maintain collective responses to achieve this. In this respect the principle of 'dementia as humanity' reminds us about wider aspects of partnership in relation to dementia. These include the role of society and communities working in partnership to provide different forms of support for people with dementia and their carers (the 'dementia-friendly community' movement is an example of this). This concept of partnership also relates to the notion of 'solidarity':

> Solidarity is the idea that we are all 'fellow travellers' and that we have duties to support and help each other and in particular those who cannot readily support themselves.
>
> (Nuffield Council on Bioethics, 2009)

It is suggested that solidarity places an obligation on society to provide support and care to people with dementia, as well as their carers, and recognizes our common humanity. We agree with this and emphasize that solidarity also supports people with dementia as potentially active participants in all the partnerships we have described. Furthermore, solidarity is demonstrated by the obligation on society to recognize dementia as a disability as well as a disease, to ensure that people benefit from the same rights as other people with disabilities.

People with dementia live their lives interdependently with families and in communities; many are able to give support as well as receive it and continue to be active participants in their communities: as employees, volunteers, members of clubs, associations, and faith communities, or activists involved in networks like the Dementia Engagement and Empowerment Project (DEEP).[3] So, *dementia as humanity* reminds us that people with dementia have relationships as citizens; practitioners who are 'duty holders' in terms of ensuring people's rights are upheld also need to be able to form partnerships with people with dementia who are 'rights-holders'. Even if a person defines their dementia as a disease, this does not mean they don't still have rights associated with dementia as a disability, thereby emphasizing the second principle of the Manifesto and the importance of VBP working in partnership with a rights-based approach. In this context dementia makes partnership more complicated but should not result in losing sight of what makes us all human.

'Nothing about us, without us' was a slogan coined by the disability movement as an assertion of people's rights to be involved in decisions about their lives. The effects of dementia, the need for partnership and support for people with dementia to express their beliefs, values, feelings, preferences, and our social interdependency led to the suggestion by one person with dementia that the slogan could be revised to incorporate these other factors: 'Nothing about us without all of us'.[4]

Partnerships and Diverse Values

Dementia as humanity encourages us to think about and treat people with dementia as people first and foremost, irrespective of the dementia; as sentient beings with values,

---

[3] www.dementiavoices.org.uk
[4] With the kind permission of Chris Roberts, speaking at Dementia Pathfinders Event, 12 July 2017, London.

preferences, and agency; and as citizens with rights. Of course, this means that partnerships in dementia care will frequently involve differences in values, as we have emphasized in this book. The purpose of VBP is to bring these differences to the surface and work with them constructively, together with other approaches integral to health and care, hence the third principle of our Manifesto, 'dementia, VBP, and rights'.

Partnerships may involve a particular set of values having priority, ranging from a more traditional practitioner-led position of 'doctor (or other professional) knows best' to 'patient power' where people with health conditions may express mistrust, disbelief or hostility towards the views of practitioners and insist on defining and directing their own care. The role of family and friends caring for people with dementia, other staff, advocates, etc., can add divergent voices and values into the partnership. While different sides may be right in certain situations, it makes the delivery of health and social care, and respect for people's rights, roles, and experiences, problematic. Reaching a consensus is often not possible. This is where VBP's principle of partnership emphasizes 'dissensus': the alternative to consensus, as we indicated for Mr Youakim in Table 11.2. We shall come back to dissensus later in the chapter.

Decision Making

Autonomous Decision Making

Understanding how we make decisions can appear somewhat in contrast to seeing people as innately social, defined in part by their relationships and, for people with dementia, as being at the centre of partnership. Many people see free will – an individual's ability to decide and act autonomously – as being a defining characteristic of what makes us human (though some strict Darwinians and many people with particular religious convictions might argue that our fate is defined more by science or a deity). This is not the place to enter into the debate about free will, but it is important to recognize how this belief and the values of autonomy and self-determination are embedded in medical ethics, health, social care values, and the law.

The concept of patient or service user autonomy is a fundamental principle of medical ethics, as well as ethical frameworks in social care. Respect for autonomy can also be found at the heart of decision making in health and social care. It is the starting place for gaining a person's consent for care or treatment; it is seen in the growing emphasis on people being encouraged to take personal responsibility for their health and for managing health conditions; and it supports the idea that people with disabilities and long-term health conditions should have choice and control over their lives and live independently insofar as possible. We are not challenging the importance of these practices in general, partly because they are genuine reflections of how we all value our own abilities of decision making and executive action – our agency. We also recognize that autonomy and self-determination for many people are the result of hard-fought struggles against oppressive, institutional cultures of care that ignored or overrode the wishes, feelings, beliefs, and values of individual service users. Our Manifesto's principles of *dementia as humanity* and *dementia as disease and disability* respect agency, and the principle of VBP in partnership with rights reflects the importance of legal frameworks designed to empower and protect individuals.

Furthermore, we are not aware of any country that has a legal framework concerning mental capacity or competency that does not locate the functional ability to make decisions anywhere other than with the individual. The principles in the Mental Capacity Act (MCA) of assuming capacity and not viewing an unwise decision as indicating a lack of capacity are examples of this. And in situations where someone is unable to make a decision, most legal frameworks require a substitute decision maker to make the decision on their behalf. On the surface, the United Nations Convention on the Rights of Persons with Disabilities (UNCRPD), which promotes a supported decision-making process as opposed to substitute decision making (discussed in more detail later), appears also to firmly locate decision-making responsibility with the individual. Decision making is about me or you, not us or them.

Yet understanding decision making in terms of an individual's autonomy and self-determination creates a tension with the notion of partnership. What is the purpose of partnership if an individual can make decisions for themselves (or on behalf of others)? Of course, many reasons provide the answer to this question, and in health and social care these often involve the need to get information, advice, guidance, experience, and expertise from others. A person being faced with a complicated and serious decision about their care or treatment for the first time may have the values that inform their decision shaped partly by the situation and the expertise of others. Deferring to the advice of professionals is common when faced with difficult and sometimes distressing decisions; 'doctor knows best' may on occasion be the preferred option for people, or they may opt to make decisions collectively with other family members. With the advent of the Internet some people may initially want to make decisions that include forms of care or treatment with a non-existent or very limited evidence base but want to discuss this with professionals. So partnerships can be found in many decision-making situations, where seeking guidance or agreement has been important. And whilst historically there has been a tendency among some health and social care professionals to assume decision-making responsibility (overriding or ignoring a person's autonomy, ability, and wish to be involved) and make the decision themselves (with or without the support of carers), more recently there has been a growing emphasis on more collective ways of decision making.

Shared Decision Making

The concept and practice of *shared decision making* is becoming increasingly common in clinical settings. Box 12.1 gives a definition of shared decision making from the UK's National Institute for Health and Care Excellence (NICE).

There is good evidence to show that shared decision making not only responds to people's wishes to be properly involved in decisions involving their care and treatment, but it also has a number of benefits in addition to those described earlier, in terms of making care, treatment, and use of services more effective (Coulter and Collins, 2011). Shared decision making is therefore an example of partnership in decision making.

Decision Making, Capacity, and Rights

Partnership in both autonomous and shared decision making becomes more problematic when the ability of someone with dementia to express their values and make decisions is compromised as a result of the cognitive impairments caused by the condition.

Again, historically, institutional and professional cultures frequently resulted in people with illnesses and disabilities involving cognitive impairments being assumed to be unable to make decisions, not being allowed to make decisions, or having their decisions

> **Box 12.1 What Is Shared Decision Making?**
>
> Shared decision making is when health professionals and patients work together. This puts people at the centre of decisions about their own treatment and care. During shared decision making, it's important that:
>
> - Care or treatment options are fully explored, along with their risks and benefits
> - Different choices available to the patient are discussed
> - A decision is reached together with a health and social care professional.
>
> **Benefits of shared decision making**
> - Both people receiving and delivering care can understand what's important to the other person
> - People feel supported and empowered to make informed choices and reach a shared decision about care
> - Health and social care professionals can tailor the care or treatment to the needs of the individual.
>
> © NICE (2018) *NICE Shared Decision Making* Available from www.nice.org.uk/about/what-we-do/our-programmes/nice-guidance/nice-guidelines/shared-decision-making. All rights reserved. Subject to Notice of rights.
>
> NICE guidance is prepared for the National Health Service in England. All NICE guidance is subject to regular review and may be updated or withdrawn. NICE accepts no responsibility for the use of its content in this product/publication.

overruled. Decisions that were made on their behalf often didn't take into account the person's wishes, feelings, beliefs, values, and preferences. The introduction of mental capacity legislation has often come about partly to protect the rights of people with cognitive impairments to make decisions for themselves whenever possible and to have clear legal processes and safeguards for decisions that have to be made on the person's behalf.

Rights are therefore of fundamental importance and inextricably linked with decision making and supporting the expression of a person's values. And one can also argue that legal frameworks for decision making emphasize partnership more than it first appears.

For example, all the key processes in the MCA (e.g. assessing capacity, making a best-interests decision) require some form of interaction between a person with dementia, who may lack capacity, and a doctor seeking their consent to treatment. This interaction in its own right involves a form of partnership so that the doctor can understand the person's values, which might inform the decisions (especially if the person's ability to make the decision has been questioned because their decision appears to be odd). But there are other elements of partnerships which support these legal processes for decision making. These are described in Box 12.2 under key parts of the MCA (more information can be found in the MCA's statutory Code of Practice (Ministry of Justice, 2007)).

Research has provided evidence of this partnership in decision making in practice. One study that looked at best-interests decisions under the MCA found that in the majority of cases decisions were made through meetings involving the person and others who knew them, multidisciplinary or joint decisions were common, and only 7 per cent of respondents to a survey (mainly practitioners) claimed to be the sole decision-maker:

> All the [best-interests decisions] I've been involved with are very much a team effort. It's not one person making a decision.
>
> (Williams et al., 2012: 63)

> **Box 12.2** MCA and Partnership in Practice
>
> **Assessment of capacity**
> - May require the views or expertise of other practitioners, family members, or others who know the person well.
>
> **Best interests decisions**
> - Consult with others in order to find out the person's views – their wishes and feelings, beliefs, values, and any other relevant factors the person might consider if they were making the decision themselves;
> - Requires involvement of an advocate in certain circumstances.
>
> **Lasting Power of Attorney, advance decisions to refuse treatment, court-appointed deputies (authorized by the court to make decisions on behalf of someone who lacks capacity)**
> - The person needs a good, trusting partnership with the individual(s) who they are authorising or expecting to make decisions on their behalf;
> - Others may be involved in creating or supervising the process for decisions to be made by someone on behalf of the person.

Yet despite the legal requirement to uphold people's rights and follow mental capacity law, whether or not this involves partnership, there is also evidence to indicate poor compliance with the law. For example, one study of 1,732 documented capacity assessments in psychiatric admissions in London showed that only 14.7 per cent explicitly demonstrated use of the MCA criteria (Brown et al., 2013). In Williams et al. (2012), of 385 reported best-interests decisions, almost 10 per cent involved cases where it was believed the person had the capacity to make the decision. The preference for consensual, collective decision making observed by the study, although commendable in many respects, was not compliant with the requirement for a single best-interests decision maker and appeared to mask an unwillingness at times by an individual to take responsibility for the decision. The same study indicated a tendency among some professionals to do a perfunctory mental capacity assessment in order to justify making a best-interests decision – a case of the tail wagging the dog.

Although these studies included but did not focus specifically on people with dementia, a report published in 2015 involving 206 people with dementia and 472 carers found that one in five people felt that professionals routinely made decisions without asking them. A majority of people (59 per cent) did not know enough about the MCA to challenge decisions made by professionals, and only 12 per cent felt that professionals supported them to make their own decisions despite it being a legal requirement (Cox, 2015).

Using the MCA as an example, legal frameworks for decision making do incorporate scope for, if not require, partnership. However, inconsistent application of the law causes difficulties in ensuring that it is a guaranteed vehicle for exporting a person's values into the decision-making processes created by those frameworks.

Supported Decision Making

A further criticism of most legal frameworks for decision making is that most are based on substitute decision making using concepts such as 'best interests' or 'benefit to the person'. If a person with dementia is assessed as being unable to make a decision, then responsibility for that decision is placed in the hands of someone else, such as a doctor, nurse, social worker, or a family member, specifically authorized to make the decision. They may have to take into account the views of the person with dementia, but they also have to consider other factors, and it is still their responsibility ultimately to make the decision.

The UNCRPD firmly opposes substitute decision making. Article 12 of the UNCRPD expresses the position that everyone has legal capacity. To deny this on the grounds of a person's disability or cognitive impairment is a fundamental contravention of a person's human rights because it would signify that a person with a disability does not have the same legal status as a person without. Instead, the UNCRPD requires a supported decision-making process to be in place, where a person's legal capacity is always respected, as much support as possible is given to help the person express his or her decision, and the 'will and preference' of the person concerned take priority in guiding the decision. A number of jurisdictions in North America, Australia, and Europe (notably the Republic of Ireland) have capacity legislation based on supported decision making (Arstein-Kerslake et al., 2017). However, when the UK government had to report on its compliance with the UNCRPD, two reports were commissioned about Article 12 compliance, and the MCA was found to be non-compliant for various reasons, including its use of substitute decision making (Burch et al., 2014; Caughey et al., 2016). So what does this all mean for practice?

Supported Decision Making – Partnership and Practice

A benefit of supported decision making is that it keeps the focus firmly on the values of the person with dementia while requiring a partnership to be formed involving practitioners, carers, advocates, and others to support the person to make or lead the decision. With Mr Youakim, those involved in the decision-making process tried to focus on what Mr Youakim would have wanted: his will and his preference.

But surely someone like Mr Youakim cannot be supported to make a decision about PEG feeding or palliative care (one might say). If he has not considered it before developing dementia and is now unable to understand the treatment interventions, communicate, or express his views about even the most basic things, how can his will and preference be identified?

This may be true, but instead of resorting to a process that runs the risk of the decision being informed by the values of the substitute decision maker, supported decision making retains a focus primarily on the values of Mr Youakim with the support of others. The outcome of the decision may be the same, but the decision-making process is a partnership involving Mr Youakim, his family, and practitioners. A supported decision-making process might not rule out disagreements about what Mr Youakim would have wanted, but it would avoid a situation where a substitute decision maker can override the views of others (including Mr Youakim). Partnership therefore supports individual decision making. Applying supported decision making is very much in keeping with person-centred practice but is also an important part of upholding the rights of people with dementia seen as a disability.

Supported Decision Making Within Substitute Decision Making

Where legal frameworks use substitute decision making, it may still be possible (and necessary) to apply a supported decision-making process, thereby upholding people's rights under the UNCRPD. Laws that include principles or processes promoting supported decision making before an assessment of capacity and potential substitute decision making takes place provide a mechanism for applying the UNCRPD approach. Assessment and best-interests decisions are the processes most familiar to practitioners using the MCA. Yet the second principle of the Act states that 'a person is not to be treated as unable to make a decision unless all practicable steps to help him [sic] to do so have been taken without success'. Although not quite the same as Article 12's definition of supported decision making in the UNCRPD, applied consistency and correctly, this principle can shift practice towards a supported decision-making approach. Where legal definitions of decision-making rights differ, it may still be possible to take a rights-based approach that is broadly in line with both definitions.

Relational Autonomy

Legal frameworks for decision making must be adhered to and, far from precluding partnership, need partnerships where a person's ability to make decisions may be compromised. But one other aspect of autonomy is also worth considering.

A collective approach to decision making is quite common in many societies and communities around the world. It also relates to the concept of 'relational autonomy', which was developed by feminist writers to signify how decision making occurs in the context of social relationships rather than by totally autonomous individuals (Ellis et al., 2011). The notion of relational autonomy is particularly important in dementia care, for both this Manifesto and VBP. An example helps illustrate what relational autonomy looks like.

Imagine a family with two young teenage children. A decision needs to be made about where to go for the family's summer holiday. In some families, responsibility for making this decision may be made by one parent alone, who does all the research on different holiday options and decides on behalf of the rest of the family. But in many families with children there will be a discussion between the parents, and the views of the children will be sought. The decision-making process will aim to be consensual, even though the ability to determine the final outcome is likely to be more limited for the children. Decision making in this context is a collective process that incorporates the views of everyone involved and occurs within social relationships.

Relational autonomy helps address the issue of people affected by dementia increasingly struggling with decision making as the condition becomes more severe. Practitioners and carers have to become more supportive and discerning about decisions involving the person with dementia. Carers in particular are an important source of information about what values would inform a person's decision about care and treatment. A person with dementia may have stated their wishes and preferences in some form of advance directive or statement or may have authorized someone else to make decisions on their behalf – both necessitate the involvement of others to ensure these wishes and preferences are followed.

Relational autonomy also reflects the principle of *dementia as humanity* – social relationships are key in defining who we are and key in how our decision making takes place. And it acknowledges that the values of everyone involved in a decision-making process influence and inform that process.

So relational autonomy can enhance supported decision making and help bridge the gap between a focus on partnership involving a person with dementia, carers, practitioners, and others and a more atomistic view of decision making focused on the individual. Recent developments in ethical thinking about dementia have emphasized the importance of relational autonomy (Nuffield Council on Bioethics, 2009). And although relational autonomy is not widely understood and is not how 'autonomy' is defined in legal frameworks, we would argue that it is a more helpful way of approaching autonomy for people whose dementia is affecting their ability to make decisions. Relational autonomy signifies partnership between the person and their carers and highlights the importance for practitioners not just to work with the person with dementia but to become part of this partnership and to support it so the person with dementia can still be central in the decision-making process.

VBP, Partnerships, and Decision Making

But VBP always draws our attention back to situations where several people with different values may be involved in decision-making processes, with different perspectives on the situation and wanting different outcomes. Alternatively, it is unclear what the values are of the person with dementia (or their carers); perhaps dementia prevents the person from fully participating in the decision-making process. Decision making in these situations is more difficult, and health or social care professionals may have to make the decision in accordance with the law. Technical expertise and experience, the need to make a decision, believing one is right, or simply ignoring the person with dementia or carers can all create power imbalances and tensions in that partnership.

The purpose of VBP is to bring differences in values to the surface and work with them constructively, together with other approaches integral to health and social care such as rights, in keeping with the third principle of our Manifesto. A partnership approach to decision making does not mean there will be agreement or consensus about the decision. This is where the concept of dissensus comes in.

Dissensus

Although all the pointers to 'good process' for VBP are important, both the concept and application of *dissensus* is absolutely key to how VBP works. Dissensus in the VBP sense is not the opposite of consensus or the same as disagreement. Dissensus means using all the other pointers in VBP to ensure that the values in play in any given situation are made explicit, there is mutual respect for those values, and as far as possible they are shared so that there can be balanced decision making. Furthermore, 'shared values' doesn't mean that everyone has to agree with them and 'sign up' to them in order to make a decision. Dissensus is where consensus may not be achievable but it's still possible to move forward without conflict or disagreement becoming an obstacle.

You might say that dissensus sounds like giving a shrug of the shoulders and saying 'I guess we will just have to agree to disagree'. There is an element of this in dissensus but it goes well beyond this sentiment. Whereas consensus is achieved by using evidence and data gradually to rule out possible decisions or actions, dissensus involves:

- Identifying and sharing all the relevant values held by different people in any given situation and keeping those values 'in play' (a bit like juggling several balls) in order that a decision is based on a dynamic balance of the relevant values according to the particular circumstances of the situation, but guided as much as possible by the values of the person with dementia, with one eye keenly on any relevant right;

- Recognizing that conflicting values do not mean that one person is right and the other is wrong or that dissensus is a bad outcome;
- For practitioners, being able to maintain 'cognitive dissonance' by holding and respecting two or more conflicting sets of values expressed by individuals on an ongoing basis for as long as they are relevant to the situation;[5]
- A willingness to make a decision based on the idea of trying one option without asserting it is necessarily the right option and that other options are wrong or should not be considered at a later date; and perhaps trickiest of all; and
- Explaining to everyone involved in language they can understand what dissensus is and how it can help provide positive solutions.

Many of the examples we have given in previous chapters illustrate dissensus, but let's consider one more that includes the difficult issue of incontinence. Urinary and faecal incontinence are quite common among people with dementia, with some estimates indicating the former may affect 38 per cent of people with dementia and the latter 27 per cent (Drennan et al., 2013). Apart from being upsetting and uncomfortable for a person with dementia, it is also likely to be distressing for family members, especially those living with the person and caring for them. Although it can be caused by a medical condition, it may also arise because the cognitive and communication impairments caused by dementia make it difficult for the person to go to the toilet or indicate they need to go to the toilet. The onset of incontinence or an increase in severity may be a trigger for carers feeling unable to continue supporting the person to live at home.

Vignette - Colin

Colin is a 59-year-old man. He is in a civil partnership with David. He was previously married to Margaret, and they have two grown-up children, Jane and Peter, but in his mid-40s Colin came out as gay. He no longer has contact with Margaret. Jane has a very good relationship with Colin and David, but Peter has always found it difficult coming to terms with Colin being gay and living with David, and his relationship with both of them is strained.

Colin used to be an engineer on cargo ships but retired when he was 55. He has drunk alcohol and smoked cigarettes in moderation all his life, but generally maintained a good level of physical fitness. When he was 38, he was diagnosed and successfully treated for prostate cancer. He said at the time if it happened again that he would prefer 'nature to take its course'. He no longer has check-ups but has said that if it returns and gets really bad, 'we will work something out together and you can always put me in a home'.

When Colin was 55 he was diagnosed with Alzheimer's disease. This led to him having to retire early and has caused him and David to have serious financial problems. Jane

---

[5] Being able to hold two contradictory truths in one's head at the same time has been described as evidence of genius by the writer F. Scott Fitzgerald and like coming to a fork in the road and taking it by the American aphorist Yogi Berra. For practitioners and carers who sensitively yet reluctantly may have to override the wishes of a service user in the short term, where this leads to a positive outcome in the long term, it may be a case of 'two wrongs can make a right' (Williamson, 2004).

was able to help them out financially. Two years later Colin fell down some steps in his garden. Although he was not seriously physically injured, he subsequently became much less fluent in speech and seemed to experience many more difficulties in remembering recent events, making decisions, and carrying out simple tasks. A subsequent visit to the doctor led to him being diagnosed with vascular dementia in addition to the Alzheimer's. The effects of the disease progressed quite rapidly, and over the last six months Colin has developed quite severe urinary incontinence that occurs on a daily basis. Colin often walks around the house saying he has to 'check the engines'; he also says he only wants to drink beer which David only lets him have in small amounts. David finds all of this upsetting and hard to deal with and feels tired and stressed caring for Colin but resists offers of help from Jane. Colin and David are visited on a regular basis by Shirley, a specialist dementia nurse.

David believes that Colin's prostate cancer may have returned and he should have further treatment which would solve the problem. The GP refers Colin for a further prostate specific antigen (PSA) test. Colin doesn't understand what the test is about, and when David takes him to the hospital he gets agitated and says he won't get out of the car, so David has to take him home. When Peter hears this, he gets angry and says to Jane that she should have taken Colin, as she would have made him see the doctor because she knows their Dad better than his 'boyfriend'. Colin's GP thinks that David is at the end of his tether and Colin should go into a care home; Jane and Peter agree, although Peter is much less concerned about David. They all point out that Colin has said he would be willing to go into a care home. David does not agree and says he would never want Colin to go into a home and that he wants to continue looking after him at home. Colin seems oblivious to the problem, gets angry if the issue is discussed in his presence, and says he is happy at home.

Shirley's Assessment
Shirley recognizes that the values and priorities of everyone involved differ. She can see how the more explicitly expressed values reflect different views on how to care for Colin but suspects that there may be more implicit, unstated values which reflect the family history and Colin coming out as gay. There is certainly no consensus on decisions about what to do. But there are no right or wrong values, which of course means that in theory Shirley has to hold a lot in her head; in reality, people will probably remind Shirley of what's important to them. There are a number of important partnerships that she must collaborate with, but these are not always straightforward. Substitute (best interests) decisions could be made, but there is scope for a supported decision-making process to be used drawing upon Colin's will and preference, as well as the views of others. Relational autonomy was expressed in Colin's statement that 'we will work something out together'.

Shirley can also see that a point may be reached where Colin will have to go into a home and acknowledges this to the GP, Jane, and Peter. However, despite Colin previously indicating that he would be willing to go into a home, Shirley doesn't believe this is currently necessary; it was expressed in relation to Colin's cancer, not dementia, and she also takes into account David's resistance to the idea, because he is the main carer.

Shirley advises David to get incontinence pads for Colin to wear but to describe them to Colin as 'protective wear a bit like some of the things you had to wear when you were at sea'. She also suggests that David encourage Colin to drink water because the engines he needs checking get very hot or to say he's 'not on the ship today' and to give him beer shandies with lots of lemonade. Colin accepts all these interventions and the explanations that David gives. Shirley also talks to David about getting support from a local carers group, sharing Colin's care more with Jane, and the possibility that Colin may have to go into a home in the future if things get much more difficult. Jane also talks to Peter about the importance of helping David in order to help their Dad, whatever views Peter has of the relationship. Shirley discusses with David supporting Colin to make decisions based on what he has said in the past, such as not trying to get him to have the PSA test in his best interests again because he clearly didn't want it and had spoken of 'letting nature take its course' (she also spoke to Peter about this). She gently reminds David of the possibility of a move to a care home, which Colin had previously given some indication that he would agree to, albeit under different circumstances. Although David is unhappy about this, he accepts it and recognizes that at some point he may no longer be able to cope.

Dissensus and the Manifesto

The example contains illustrations of what we have discussed in this chapter. Dissensus and the other themes in this chapter provide a viable and constructive way of achieving balanced decision making in any given situation that can effectively address disagreements and incorporate the different values in play, rather than rejecting or subordinating them.

We also recognize that the first two principles of our Manifesto, *dementia as humanity* and *dementia as disease and disability*, do not necessarily convert easily into actual practice. A person with dementia may say things that are rude or offensive, or become agitated and aggressive. Carers may express anger, frustration, or exhaustion. Limitations on resources may mean that respecting the rights and decisions of a person with dementia is problematic. The effects of someone's dementia may mean that medical interventions are necessary which are in conflict with supporting them as a person with a disability.

The benefit of dissensus in situations like these is that it shines a spotlight on the different values in play, and is an important example of how the third principle of our Manifesto, *dementia, VBP, and rights*, can be used to make the other two principles make more sense. Both principles contain an element of dissensus. Dementia as humanity incorporates a focus on people as autonomous decision makers, but also relationally in partnerships with loved ones and families, with friends, practitioners and services, communities, and the *polis*. Dementia as disease and disability acknowledges both the individual experience of a health condition that can be distressing and the wish for personal care and treatment, but also how dementia can be considered a disability, requiring a collective response from the wider society. And of course, dissensus can be important in enabling values identified and expressed through VBP to be balanced with values arising from a rights-based approach where there is not always agreement.

To illustrate how dissensus connects with the Manifesto's principles, let's go back to Colin and think about two aspects of the approach taken to support him involving both VBP and a rights-based approach.

- Dissensus may involve practitioners and carers accepting risks which may feel uncomfortable but respects the decisions, values, will, preference, and rights of the person with dementia. There were risks involved with Colin staying at home and not having the PSA test, but the decisions involved were in line with a supported decision-making approach that respected Colin's will and preference. This couldn't be done simply as an assertion of Colin's rights but needed to recognize him as a person with wishes and feelings, expressing agency, and as part of a negotiated process with David, Jane, Peter, and the GP who also had wishes, feelings, beliefs, and values: *dementia as humanity*.

- Dissensus may require using a range of interventions aimed at understanding and potentially 'going along with' values expressed through a factually untrue 'reality' or belief held by the person with dementia, even if there is only a very limited evidence base for the approach. The reason for this approach is that it appears to maximize the person's wellbeing or enable the person to cope with his or her situation. In Colin's case this involved going along with his intermittent belief that he was back working in his seaman days to address his incontinence and encourage him to drink more. The approach required David and others to adapt to Colin's beliefs, accommodating his dementia as a disability, as much as it attempted to address Colin's dementia as a disease that had resulted in both his incontinence and dehydration.

Dissensus about Dissensus

Dissensus and the other pointers in VBP do not provide the answers to every difficult situation involving values in dementia care. In previous chapters we have described lots of examples of these, but as a reminder here are a few, described in brief statements from different people's perspectives:

- I'm not unwell.
- I don't have dementia.
- I don't need help.
- I want this kind of support/care/treatment [which is unavailable].
- I know what's best for my husband/wife/spouse/partner and it's not that.
- We must overrule the wishes of the person with dementia and/or their carers to make the person safe.
- We must respect the autonomy and wishes of the person at all times.

There are no easy solutions in these situations, and each one has to be dealt with in its own right. But we believe that the principles of our Manifesto and using an approach incorporating dissensus and the other pointers of VBP provide important ways of approaching and responding to situations like these when they arise. Partnerships and decision making are about people and will inevitably at times be the source of disagreements – dissensus offers a way of dealing with these constructively. The complexities of dementia, values, evidence, rights, and limitations on knowledge require the use of everyone's experience and expertise but also humility in the face of uncertainty – this may be frustrating, but it is also a reality.

But going back to the tricky situations we've described in the bullet points earlier, don't dissensus and the Manifesto just make it all too complicated? No! It just means that in a decision-making situation involving a person with dementia, especially where the person has difficulties expressing their views or making a decision, we must not allow ourselves to become fixated on certain values, evidence, rights, or views of one person (including our own views), whether it's the view of the person with dementia, carers, or other practitioners, without considering all the relevant values, evidence, rights, or views of others. Dementia as humanity and dementia as disease and disability just require us to start by seeing everyone, whether they have dementia or not, as people first, and as being open to all the possibilities for understanding dementia in any given situation. Dementia, VBP, and rights is a further reminder of the importance of always having this open, empathic, and inclusive approach. Dementia care and practice that arise from this may not be easy or consensual but are likely to be much more inclusive and respectful.

Conclusion

Partnership in decision making is the element of VBP where values are most evident in everyday practice. Partnerships and decision making involve people, as individuals but also in relationships with others. There are bound to be differences in values; dissensus is key in providing a positive framework to accommodate these differences, make decisions, and move forward in partnership, providing care, treatment, and support. It provides a practical way of applying the principles of our Manifesto in difficult situations that arise. We conclude with two quotes from people with dementia that describe very different perspectives on the condition: one as almost an intrinsic part of the person, the other as an objective disease. Dissensus enables us to work with both:

> I become convinced that I am right in the face of explanations which attempt to prove to me that I am wrong. I resent and resist these attempts and experience them as oppressive. I am capable of being lucid, rational and I can still exercise good judgment some of the time. Other states of consciousness have often left me mistrustful of my own grasp on what is real as well as anxious about the decisions I need to make for myself. However I find myself mostly much more mistrustful of others making these decisions about me without me. I mostly feel anxious with good reason but sometimes I must admit my anxiety is misplaced. My overall forgetfulness feeds into my anxiety because I cannot be sure whether what I remember is real or imagined. An example is thinking about something but then imagining that other people were present for a conversation about this. Subsequently they deny the conversation because it didn't take place. I am frequently accused of false memories. My caregivers, family and friends frequently assume they know when I am confused. They think they know what I am thinking. I get angry about this.

> They are frightening. I understand them as an aberration of normal thinking due to brain disease ... they are separate to who I am and I cannot use 'my' mind during an onslaught ... I have to wait for it to take its course.

(Williamson and Kirtley, 2016: 38)

References

Adams, T., Holman, M., and Mitchell, G. (2003). Multidisciplinary teamworking. In J. Keady, C. Clarke, and T. Adams, eds., *Community Mental Health Nursing and Dementia Care.* Maidenhead and Philadelphia: Open University Press, 33–44.

Arstein-Kerslake, A., Watson, J., Browning, M., Martinis, J. ,and Blanck, P (2017). Future directions in supported decision-making. *Disability Studies Quarterly* 37, 1. http://dsq-sds.org/article/view/5070/4549 (accessed 22 January 2018).

Brown, P., Tulloch, A., Mackenzie, C., et al. (2013). Assessment of mental capacity in psychiatric inpatients: A retrospective cohort study. *BMC Psychiatry* **13**, https://link.springer.com/article/10.1186/1471-244X-13-115 (accessed 22 January 2018).

Burch, M., Jutten, T., Martin, W., and Michalowski, S. (2014). *Achieving CRPD Compliance*. Essex: University of Essex, The Essex Autonomy Project. https://autonomy.essex.ac.uk/wp-content/uploads/2017/01/EAP-Position-Paper-FINAL.pdf (accessed 22 January 2018).

Caughey, C., Hempsey, A., Martin, W., et al. (2016). *Three Jurisdictions Report: Towards Compliance with CRPD Art. 12 in Capacity/Incapacity Legislation across the UK*. Essex: University of Essex, The Essex Autonomy Project. https://autonomy.essex.ac.uk/wp-content/uploads/2017/01/EAP-3J-Final-Report-2016.pdf (accessed 22 January 2018).

Chakkalackal, L. (2014). The value of peer support on cognitive improvement amongst older people living with dementia. *Research, Policy and Planning* **31**, 127–41. http://ssrg.org.uk/members/files/2015/07/Chakkalackal_v2.pdf (accessed 22 January 2018).

Coulter, A., and Collins, A. (2011). *Making Shared Decision-Making a Reality*. London: The King's Fund. www.kingsfund.org.uk/sites/default/files/Making-shared-decision-making-a-reality-paper-Angela-Coulter-Alf-Collins-July-2011_0.pdf (accessed 22 January 2018).

Drennan, V., Rait, G., Cole, L., Grant, R., and Iliffe, S. (2013). The prevalence of incontinence in people with cognitive impairment or dementia living at home: A systematic review. *Neurology and Urodynamics* **32**, 314–24. http://eprints.kingston.ac.uk/23984/1/Drennan-V-23984.pdf (accessed 22 January 2018).

Cox, S. (2015). Decision-making and dementia – how well does the Mental Capacity Act serve people living with the condition? *Elder Law Journal* **5**(1), 74–83.

Ellis, C., Hunt, M. R., and Chambers-Evans, J. (2011). Relational autonomy as an essential component of patient-centred care. *International Journal of Feminist Approaches to Bioethics* **4**, 79–101. www.mcgill.ca/biomedicalethicsunit/files/biomedicalethicsunit/ellshunt-chambersrelationalautonomyijfab2011.pdf (accessed 22 January 2018).

Firth, G., and Barber. M. (2011). *Using Intensive Interaction with a Person with a Social or Cognitive Impairment*. London: Jessica Kingsley Publishers.

Frost, L. A., and Bondy, A. S. (1994). *PECS: The Picture Exchange Communications System Training Manual*. Cherry Hill, NJ: Pyramid Educational Consultants.

Luker, K. A., Austin, L., Caress, A., and Hallett, C. E. (2008). The importance of 'knowing the patient': Community nurses' constructions of quality in providing palliative care. *Journal of Advanced Nursing* **31**(4), 775–82.

McCabe, R., and Priebe, S. (2004). The therapeutic relationship in the treatment of severe mental illness: A review of methods and findings. *International Journal of Social Psychiatry* **50**(2), 115–28.

Midgley, M. (2010). *The Solitary Self: Darwin and the Selfish Gene*. Durham: Acumen.

Ministry of Justice. (2007). *Mental Capacity Act 2005 Code of Practice*. London: HMSO. www.gov.uk/government/uploads/system/uploads/attachment_data/file/497253/Mental-capacity-act-code-of-practice.pdf (accessed 22 January 2018).

Miranda-Castillo, C., Woods, B., and Orrell, M. (2010). People with dementia living alone: What are their needs and what kind of support are they receiving? *International Psychogeriatrics*, **22**, 607–17. www.cambridge.org/core/journals/international-psychogeriatrics/article/people-with-dementia-living-alone-what-are-their-needs-and-what-kind-of-support-are-they-receiving/6AE02C5BA023C45A8A5A79F6A30B6963 (accessed 22 January 2018).

Nuffield Council on Bioethics. (2009). *Dementia: Ethical Issues*. London: Nuffield Council on Bioethics. http://nuffieldbioethics.org/wp-content/uploads/2014/07/Dementia-report-Oct-09.pdf (accessed 22 January 2018).

Reynolds, B. (2009). Developing therapeutic one-to-one relationships. In P. Barker, ed., *Psychiatric and Mental Health Nursing*. London: Edward Arnold Publishers.

Struble, L. M., Kavanagh, J., and Blazek, M. (2013). Services for people with moderate dementia. In H. de Waal, C. Lyketsos, D. Ames, and J. O'Brien, eds., *Designing and Delivering Dementia Services*. Oxford: Wiley Blackwell, 73–89.

Thompsell, A. (2011). Support to care homes. In T. Dening and A. Milne, eds., *Mental Health and Care Homes*. Oxford: Oxford University Press, 221–36.

Williams, V., Boyle, G., Jepson, M., et al. (2012). *Making Best Interests Decisions:*

People and Processes. London: Mental Health Foundation. www.mentalhealth .org.uk/sites/default/files/BIDS_ report_24-02-12_FINAL1.pdf (accessed 22 January 2018).

Williamson, T. (2004). Can two wrongs make a right? *Philosophy, Psychiatry, & Psychology* 11, 159–63. https://muse.jhu.edu/ article/173772 (accessed 22 January 2018).

Williamson, T., and Kirtley, A. (2016). *Dementia Truth Inquiry. Review of Evidence*. London: Mental Health Foundation. www .mentalhealth.org.uk/sites/default/files/ dementia-truth-enquiry-roe_0.pdf (accessed 22 January 2018).

Conclusion

In the *Economic and Philosophic Manuscripts of 1844*, Karl Marx wrote the following:

> [M]y *own* existence *is* social activity, and therefore that which I make of myself, I make of myself for society and with the consciousness of myself as a social being.
>
> (Marx, 1932: 44).[1]

The idea that we are interconnected and interdependent social beings is one that underpins our Manifesto. As we said at the beginning, a manifesto is a public declaration. Our declaration is encapsulated by three slogans, which have acted as our principles:

- *Dementia as humanity* – the thought that dementia is a unique touchstone for understanding the human condition;
- *Dementia as disease and disability* – which emphasizes the rights of people living with dementia to all the usual benefits of citizenship, whilst also recognizing its effects as a physical disease on people's lives;
- *Dementia, VBP, and rights* – according to which VBP and an awareness of rights provides an essential framework for providing support, care, and treatment to people with dementia, their families, and their friends.

All three principles are rooted in the thought that as human beings in the world, we are quintessentially social. The implications of this can be generalized. We see this increasingly in the globalization of the world, where our actions in one part of the world are not irrelevant to people (as well as animals and plants) on the far side of the world. And what we say and do here, now, can be known immediately elsewhere. Dementia is a global issue for all of humanity. But it's not just something that other people have. It's a way of being which is both unique and yet no different from any other. Each person is individual, but

---

[1] Inevitably, this passage is translated differently elsewhere. For instance, in Marx, K. (1961). *Selected Writings in Sociology and Social Philosophy*, 2nd edn (eds. T. B. Bottomore and M. Rubel; trans. T. B. Bottomore), Harmondsworth: Penguin Books, page 91, it appears as follows: 'My *own* existence *is* a social activity. For this reason, what I myself produce, I produce for society and with the consciousness of acting like a social being'. For our purposes, the idea of *making something of ourselves* is more pertinent than the idea of *economic productivity*, which might help to reassure some readers that, for the purposes of this book, we are not interested in Marxism as such, nor then in Marxist revolution! But some of the insights of Karl Marx (and Friedrich Engels) remain inspiring and, for our purposes, can support the need for a type of revolution at a personal and social level in terms of how we think about and live with dementia. This is not to deny that the inspiration for such a revolution could equally come from other sources, from religions or from humanism, for instance.

our individuality is social. The problems that confront people living with dementia are, surely, problems for us all. This is captured by notions of solidarity and citizenship, which suggest our membership of the *polis*, where this means not just a particular state but the whole of society. Furthermore, our standing as citizens, where this also gestures at diverse and shared interests, entails some sense of our rights: rights which exist in part to protect the things that we value.

Because dementia can have profound effects on a person's self-knowledge and awareness of what is reality, it can also require others to reflect on who they are as individuals in relation to a person with dementia. Different realities may be 'in the moment' or last for much longer but may well involve expressions of both shared and divergent values. So how we deal with values – VBP being one process, but one that has been considered and found to be useful – particularly when they are diverse, is crucial for us all if we are to live and enable others to live in a just and compassionate world.

The process of VBP, with its emphasis on clinical and practice skills (which includes good communication), on professional relationships, on evidence as well as values, and on partnership, is also about recognizing the social basis of practice. The emphasis on the importance of scientific evidence might seem at odds with this statement, except that the point of this emphasis in VBP is that it matches, is a complement to, the equally important emphasis on values. Science needs to be seen as a social endeavour. Scientists are not cut off from society; they are part of it. As a result, they must confront or be aware of the social and ethical implications of their work. Without this input, science is undoubtedly dangerous. But cognizant of its ethical responsibilities, science is a potential force for good. In health care and social practice, underpinned by good science, evaluative judgements are inevitable, and the awareness of this that VBP encourages is therefore crucial. But as we've been at pains to emphasize throughout, VBP must be supplemented by an overt acknowledgement of rights. The rights of citizens with dementia may well push back against the inclinations of others and – as we have seen in the discussion of the difference between substituted and supported decision making – will change attitudes and practice.

This brings us, then, to our final thoughts. A manifesto is a public proclamation, but proclamations are not intended to be just words. They are intended to have an effect. We should be (and are) modest in our expectations of the effects of our Manifesto. Modesty is required because, after all, we are simply part of a movement which has emerged, and is emerging, and would emerge irrespective of this book. Nevertheless, we would contend that our Manifesto should encourage this movement, which can be conceived of as a revolution. It's a person-centred, rights-based, values-aware revolution in connection with dementia which accepts difference, as well as divergent views.

It can be sensed in the academic literature. From important papers, such as those produced over many years by Dr Ruth Bartlett (e.g. Bartlett and O'Connor, 2007; Bartlett, 2014), whose work can be summed up to some extent by the quote on her webpage at the University of Southampton: 'A citizenship lens has a lot to offer the dementia care field' (see www.southampton.ac.uk/healthsciences/about/staff/rlb1r10.page), to the book that is being completed as we write by Dr Suzanne Cahill from Trinity College Dublin, *Dementia and Human Rights* (Cahill, in press). (We have already mentioned, in Chapter 11, the paper by Shakespeare et al., 2017.) It can be sensed, too, at the level of grassroots activism by people with dementia (and carers) and government policy, where in England there is currently a move to extend the use of the 'blue badge' scheme to people with 'invisible' disabilities, such as dementia and autism. (The blue badge scheme allows people with disabilities to park their cars in restricted areas.) This has been partly the result of campaigning by groups led by people with dementia that are part of the Dementia Engagement & Empowerment Project (DEEP) network mentioned in Chapter 2. It also follows the extension of the Prime Minister's Challenge on Dementia mentioned in Chapter 2, with its emphasis on dementia-friendly communities, which (in essence) promoted a notion of citizenship for people living with dementia.

In addition, this revolution can really be sensed at the personal level. People with dementia are becoming more assertive of their rights and of their continuing standing as citizens who have a voice, or more correctly, many voices (https://dementiadiaries .org). Indeed, Keith Oliver, who has kindly read and commented on our Manifesto, has also addressed the United Nations Committee on the Rights of Persons with Disabilities. His feedback from this experience demonstrates the progress made, in that people with dementia have been included amongst those with disabilities, which means that the rights afforded to people living with dementia are in step with the rights of people with other disabilities (https://dementiadiaries.org/entry/5087/reporting-back-after-the-un-committee-on-rights-of-persons-with-disabilities). But it also shows that there is much more work to be done, because the committee was seemingly poorly informed about dementia. In a sense, then, dementia could be seen as being at the cutting edge, if not leading current debates about disability rights. It was also apparent that groups representing other disabilities were better organized and politically savvier than Keith and his supporters. People with dementia have also written about their experiences of dementia, from America (Davis, 1989), to the UK (Saints and De Frene, 2014; Mitchell, 2018), to Australia (Swaffer, 2016), and elsewhere. Such writing, and there is much more, both provides insight into what it is like to live with dementia and advocates for those who do live with it.

In the UK, the DEEP network supports groups 'to try to change services and policies that affect the lives of people with dementia' (http://dementiavoices.org.uk). It is another manifestation of the commitment on the part of people living with dementia to change the world for the better, to assert their rights as citizens who are still able and keen to engage with society, and to participate in decisions about matters which concern them.

Our values reflect who we are. Societal values shape our lives and create pressure to conform, but our civil and human rights support and protect our ability to live together in the ways that we wish, even where these may not conform. This is true for us all. It must also be true for people living with dementia. Our Manifesto is about living together as citizens of the world, with rights and values. Our hope is that this Manifesto will feed into the *zeitgeist*, the spirit of the age, which places the values and rights of people with dementia centre stage. After all: 'They have a world to win' (Marx and Engels, 1967: 121).

References

Bartlett, R. (2014). Citizenship in action: The lived experiences of citizens with dementia who campaign for social change. *Disability and Society* 29, 1291–304.

Bartlett, R., and O'Connor, D. (2007). From personhood to citizenship: Broadening the lens for dementia practice and research. *Journal of Aging Studies*, **21**, 107–18.

Cahill, S. (in press). *Dementia and Human Rights.* Bristol, UK, and Chicago, USA: Policy Press.

Davis, R. (1989). *My Journey into Alzheimer's Disease: Helpful Insights for Family and Friends.* Wheaton, IL: Tyndale House.

Marx, K. (1932). *Economic and Philosophic Manuscripts of 1844.* Translated by Martin Milligan from the German text, revised by Dirk J. Struik, contained in Marx/Engels, Gesamtausgabe, Abt. 1, Bd. 3. Sourced from: www.marxists.org/ archive/marx/works/download/pdf/

Economic-Philosophic-Manuscripts-1844
.pdf [last accessed 31 January, 2018].

Marx, K., and Engels, F. (1967). *The Communist Manifesto* (translated by Samuel Moore and first published in 1888). Harmondsworth: Penguin Books.

Mitchell, W. (2018). *Somebody I Used to Know*. London: Bloomsbury.

Saints, M. J., and De Frene, B. (2014). *Welcome to Our World: A Collection of Life Writings* *by People Living with Dementia*. Edited by Liz Jennings. Fareham: Forget Me Not Publications.

Shakespeare, T., Zeilig, H., and Mittler, P. (2017). Rights in mind: Thinking differently about dementia and disability. *Dementia* 0(0), 1–14. doi: 10.1177/1471301217701506

Swaffer, K. (2016). *What the Hell Happened to My Brain? Living Beyond Dementia*. London and Philadelphia: Jessica Kingsley.

Index